Griffiths'
Sport Supplement Review

DR PETER GRIFFITHS qualified as a doctor from the University of London where he was a multi award winning graduate and winner of the prestigious St. George's Dermatology Prize. He also holds a Masters degree in Esthetic Medicine from the University of Cordoba in Spain. After qualifying he gained further experience in psychiatry, cardiology and urology and in addition to being the author of several books he also writes for the Lance Armstrong Foundation as an expert on sports supplements and nutrition. Regular articles and updates on these subjects can be found on his website at -

www.doctorpg.org

Griffiths'
Sport Supplement Review

Dr. P J Griffiths BA (Hons) MBBS MSc

Published by Dr. P J Griffiths

Copyright © Peter J Griffiths 2011

First published 2011

ISBN 978-0-9569195-0-2

e-ISBN 978-0-9569195-1-9

Permissions may be sought from drgriffiths@doctorpg.org

www.doctorpg.org

Contents

Note on expanded contents: many supplements have several different names. To aid the reader in identifying a supplement an expanded contents list is provided which includes all the alternative names for each supplement.

Introduction

The sports supplement market is huge and growing larger every year. A recent survey revealed 44% of men now use some kind of specific sport nutrition product to support their training. In 2010 spending on sports nutrition products was over $5 billion in the US and $2 billion in Europe.

A look at any sports supplement store or web site will quickly reveal a huge variety of sport supplements with various performance enhancing claims and it seems as if a new one appears virtually every week.

But what exactly is a sport supplement and how can sports people, consumers, professional trainers and medical professionals evaluate their effectiveness and safety?

There is no strict definition of a sport supplement. A sport supplement can be considered as any supplement taken as an ergogenic aid. That is, a supplement intended to improve sport performance, exercise capacity and training adaptations. In other words it helps an individual to perform better and recover faster.

As a result of this wide definition sports supplements may be composed of a wide variety of ingredients including food components such as carbohydrate, protein, fat or vitamins and minerals. They may also contain herbs or various other plant extracts, or other metabolic intermediates such as amino acids.

This immediately reveals a problem for those seeking reliable information about the efficacy or safety of sports supplements. Due to the wide variety of ingredients, information may have to be sought from a wide variety of sources. Information may be found for some supplements in reference works about dietary and food supplements. For others sources regarding herbal and natural medicines will need to be consulted. For yet others research in scientific or medical textbooks and journals will need to be consulted.

Anyone who has attempted to find information about sports supplements in such sources will also immediately recognize another problem. Such sources frequently concentrate on the health benefits or medicinal properties of supplements and herbs and little information is given specifically regarding the use of such compounds for improving sports performance.

In addition, while short abstracts or summaries of scientific studies are often available for free on sites such as Pubmed access to full studies often requires subscriptions to medical or scientific journals which most people simply do not have. Furthermore such studies can be written in confusing scientific jargon which may make them difficult to understand for lay people who are not experts in the field.

It is these problems which I aim to address in this book. By providing a rigorous scientific evaluation of the evidence for the most commonly used sports supplements without distracting the readers' attention with unnecessary information about general health benefits or the use of individual supplements for particular health conditions.

I have attempted to make this book as useful as possible to both sports people and medical and health professionals. I have tried to make the explanations understandable and readable to lay people while also including full scientific referencing so that those who wish to check facts or do their own research can do so. All references are provided in the

Dr. P J Griffiths

full Vancouver referencing system standard in scientific journals.

Evaluating supplements
– the star system

How has this book and how should sports people and health professionals in general evaluate the evidence for a particular sports supplement? To a large extent this is based on common sense. Studies using live animals or people (*in vivo* studies) generally provide better information than studies which test substances in a test tube (*in vitro* studies). Studies which use humans are more useful than studies using rats. Studies which are designed to specifically test the effect of a supplement on sports performance, or muscle growth in healthy individuals for example, will provide more useful information than a study which looks at the effect of a supplement on sick people. Studies using 1000 people are much more convincing than studies using 5 people.

Then we can also look at the design of the study. The gold standard is known as a double blind placebo controlled trial. This means that the substance being tested is tested on two groups, one receiving the real substance and the other receiving an inert placebo. Neither the test subjects nor the scientists themselves know who is receiving the real treatment or a placebo (hence double blind).

Finally we should consider where and how the results of studies are published. Are they published in prestigious scientific journals or do they appear in lesser known journals where they will be subject to less scrutiny? Is the full study published allowing other researchers to fully evaluate the results or is only a summary or abstract published?

When supplements appear claiming to be supported by scientific studies but the studies have only been published as abstracts in obscure journals we should be suspicious. We should be doubly cautious if the studies have been financed by a supplement company or the researchers have a financial interest in the supplement such as holding the patent or shares in a company marketing the supplement. Most scientific journals require scientists to declare such conflicts of interest in the footnotes to published studies.

Of course I need to sound a note of caution here regarding scientific studies. Just because a supplement is not supported by any studies does not necessarily mean it is useless. A supplement may be too new for studies to have been carried out. For other supplements studies may never be done. Studies are expensive to carry out and unless a compound being tested is capable of being patented and providing a financial return few companies are likely to bother financing research.

But just because specific studies are not available does not mean we cannot use our judgement to evaluate a supplement. We can still consider if the claims made for a supplement are in accordance with known principals of human physiology and pharmacology. Or are the claims being made outlandish and fantastical? We should be wary of any product claiming results equivalent to anabolic steroids or produced by companies which have a history of over-hyped marketing.

As you go through this book you will realize that there are in fact very few supplements which have 100% convincing evidence of effectiveness. Evidence is on a continuum from poor to better for the majority of supplements and which ones a sports person decides to invest their time and money in will be a personal choice based on personal circumstances and budget. Some people will not want to spend their money on anything but the most proven products. Others with money to spare or who simply wish to experiment may decide to try products with less evidence supporting them.

In order to help the reader evaluate the evidence for a particular supplement I have classified all the supplements in this book by a star system. This is not meant to be a rigorous scientific classification but is a rough guide to the level of evidence which in my professional opinion supports a supplement. The system assigns a value as outlined below from one to five with one star being the lowest score and five stars being the highest or best score.

5 Star : The supplement's claimed benefit has been demonstrated in humans in several large studies and there is a recognised body of evidence for its effectiveness.

4 Star : The supplement's claimed benefit has been demonstrated in humans in one or more large studies or a number of small studies.

Or; The supplement's mode of action (e.g. increase in testosterone levels) has been demonstrated in humans in several large studies although its proposed benefit (e.g. increased muscle mass) has either not been demonstrated or not tested.

3 Star : The supplement's claimed benefit or mode of action has been demonstrated in humans in one or more small studies.

2 Star : The supplement's claimed benefit or mode of action has only been demonstrated in animal or *in vitro* (test tube) cell studies.

1 Star : Only anecdotal or manufacturers information exists regarding the supplements mode of action or claimed benefit in humans.

Doses

The following is a brief explanation of the metric system of dosing used throughout this book.

One milligram (1mg) is one thousandth of a gram (1g) and one microgram (which can be written either as 1mcg or 1µg) is one millionth of a gram.

Therefore –

1g = 1000mg
1mg = 1000mcg

International units or IU is an internationally recognized method of measuring the quantity of compounds based on their biological activity. It is usually used for fat soluble vitamins such as vitamins A, D, E and K and medications such as some hormones and vaccines.

As better methods of measuring many of these compounds have been developed the IU system is being replaced with measures in mg or mcg in many cases although the IU system is still in wide use particularly for vitamin E.

Since the biological activity of each compound is different the conversion rate of IU to mg is also different for each compound. For example 1IU of vitamin E = 0.671mg while 1IU of vitamin A = 0.3mcg.

Important information – please read !

Nothing in this book is intended to be a substitute for medical advice or treatment. Anyone with a medical condition or taking any kind of medication whether prescribed or over the counter should consult a suitably qualified medical practitioner before taking any kind of supplement.

This also applies to anyone who is pregnant or planning to get pregnant or anyone who is breast feeding.

Information on doses in the sections of this book titled "Commonly used doses" are not to be taken as a recommendation to use the doses mentioned or that a particular dose is safe. Always adhere to the recommended maximum doses indicated by the manufacturer of your supplement. Consult a suitably qualified medical practitioner if you are in any doubt.

Information in this book on the safety and interactions of the supplements covered is intended to be a general guide but is not an exhaustive list of all possible interactions nor is it a guarantee of the safety of any particular supplement. If you are in any doubt you must consult a suitably qualified medical practitioner.

The information in this book is intended for the use of adults over the age of 18. Children under the age of 18 should not use supplements unless on the recommendation or under the supervision of a suitably qualified medical practitioner.

A – Z Guide

Achyranthes

Other names

Chirchita
Niu Xi

Various species of achyranthes exist including arborescens, aspera and bidentata.

Star rating

2

What is it?

A genus of plants (perennial) from the Amaranthaceae family used in traditional Chinese and Indian medicine.

Claimed benefits

Weight loss

Mode of Action

Diuretic and increased activity of the thyroid gland causing increased serum levels of the thyroid hormones T3 and T4.

Effectiveness

The diuretic activity of achyranthes has only been

demonstrated in rats in a study reported in the Indian Journal of Pharmacology (1). The thyroid stimulating action has similarly only been demonstrated in seven rats in an Indian study reported in The Journal of Ethnopharmacology (2).

Commonly used dosages

Achyranthes is usually included as part of a proprietary formulation in commercial sport supplement preparations with the exact quantity of the substance not listed in the ingredients.

It is not usually sold as a stand alone supplement. In the study cited above demonstrating increased thyroid hormone levels in rats an amount of extract equivalent to 200 mg/kg body weight was used.

Safety

There is one report of a man suffering unconsciousness from a slow heart rate after ingesting a large quantity of achyranthes (3).

Interactions

None known.

References

1. Gupta SS, Verma SC, Ram AK, Tripathi RM. Diuretic effect of the saponin of Achyranthes aspera (Apamarga). Ind J Pharmacol. 1972;4:208-14
2. Tahiliani P, Kar A. Achyranthes aspera elevates thyroid hormone levels and decreases hepatic lipid peroxidation in male rats. J Ethnopharmacol. 2000;71(3):527-32

3. Han ST, Un CC. Cardiac toxicity caused by Achyranthes aspera. Vet Hum Toxicol. 2003;45(4):212-3

Agaricus

Other names

Agarikusutake
Almond Mushroom
Brazil Mushroom
Cogumelo de Deus
Cogumelo do Sol
Himematsutake
Kawariharatake
Mandelpilz

Star rating

2

What is it?

Agaricus is a genus of mushroom which contains hundreds of species. The most commonly known are Agaricus bisporus, Agaricus campestris, and Agaricus subrufescens (formerly known as Agaricus blazei). It is Agaricus subrufescens which is usually promoted as a medicinal agent and claimed to be useful in the treatment of cancer, diabetes, high cholesterol and heart disease.

Claimed benefits

Weight loss.

Mode of Action

Increases secretion of adiponectin (also known as Acrp30, AdipoQ and apm-1) a protein hormone secreted by adipocytes (fat cells). The exact function of adiponectin is unclear but it appears to reduce levels of plasma glucose and free fatty acids by increasing cellular sensitivity to the effects of insulin and an acute increase in fatty acid oxidation (burning of fat for energy) by muscle tissue (1).

Effectiveness

The ability of exogenously administered adinopectin to increase insulin sensitivity and regulate fatty acid oxidation has been demonstrated in animal studies (1), (2), (3) but not in human studies. However studies in humans indicate that levels of adinopectin are inversely correlated with bodyweight, i.e. obese individuals have lower levels of adinopectin and slimmer individuals have higher levels of adinopectin (4), (5). But a causal relationship has not been proven i.e. it is not certain whether it is the level of adinopectin which causes changes in bodyweight.

The ability of agaricus to directly cause an increase in plasma levels of adinopectin has not been demonstrated. However one reasonably large Chinese study (6) has shown that agaricus in combination with diabetes medication can improve insulin sensitivity in diabetic individuals (type II diabetes) and this was accompanied by a 20% increase in plasma adiponectin concentration. Nevertheless the ability of agaricus to cause weight loss in healthy individuals has not been tested.

Commonly used dosages

Agaricus is usually included as part of a proprietary

formulation in commercial sport supplement preparations with the exact quantity of the substance not listed in the ingredients.

When sold as a stand alone supplement capsules of 400 to 600mg are common with recommended doses being one to three capsules a day.

In the Chinese study which showed an improvement in insulin sensitivity and 20% increase in adiponectin levels, the test subjects took 1500mg a day.

Safety

No known safety issues.

Interactions

May potentiate the effect of diabetes medication and cause lower than normal blood glucose levels (6).

References

1. Fruebis J, Tsao T, Javorschi S, Ebbets-Reed D, Erickson MRS, Yen FT, Bihain BE, Lodish HF. Proteolytic cleavage product of 30-kDa adipocyte complement-related protein increases fatty acid oxidation in muscle and causes weight loss in mice. Proc Natl Acad Sci U.S.A. 2001;98(4):2005-10
2. Berg AH, Combs TP, Scherer PE. ACRP30/adiponectin: an adipokine regulating glucose and lipid metabolism. Trends Endocrinol Metab 2002; 13(2):84-89
3. Qi Y, Takahashi N, Hileman SM, Patel HR, Berg AH, Pajvan UB. *et al.* Adiponectin acts in the brain to decrease body weight. Nat Med 2004;10:524-529

4. Reinehr T, Roth C, Menke T, Andler W. Adiponectin before and after Weight Loss in Obese Children. J Clin Endocrinol Metab. 2004;89(8): 3790-3794

5. Valsamakis G. McTernanb PG, Chettyb R, Al Daghrib N, Fielda A, Hanifab W. *et al.* Modest weight loss and reduction in waist circumference after medical treatment are associated with favorable changes in serum adipocytokines . Metabolism. 2004;53(4):430-434

6. Hsu CH, Liao YL, Lin SC, *et al.* The mushroom Agaricus Blazei Murill in combination with metformin and gliclazide improves insulin resistance in type 2 diabetes: a randomized, double-blinded, and placebo-controlled clinical trial. J Altern Complement Med 2007;13:97-102.

Agmatine

Other names

1-Amino-4-guanidobutane
2-(4-aminobutyl)guanidine
Agmathine
Agmatine sulfate
Argmatine
N-4-aminobutylguanidine

Star Rating

2

What is it?

Decarboxylated arginine produced in bacteria, plants and invertebrates. It is produced in mammalian brains and stored in other organs (1). From animal studies agmatine appears to be a neurotransmitter involved in various metabolic processes.

Claimed benefits

If one were to believe some supplement manufacturers, agmatine can be regarded as a miracle substance which can do just about anything. However the main claimed benefits are an anabolic action, improvement in body composition (more lean muscle and less fat tissue) and analgesic action.

Mode of Action

Anabolic action and improvement in body composition via:

- Increased testosterone levels via stimulation of pituitary luteinizing hormone and hypothalamic luteinizing hormone-releasing hormone.
- Increased pituitary human growth hormone (GH) release.
- Increased insulin release from islet cells.

Analgesic action: mode of action unclear, perhaps via NMDA receptor antagonism.

Effectiveness

The ability of agmatine to stimulate release of luteinizing hormone from the pituitary gland has only been demonstrated in rats when agmatine was injected directly into their brains (2).

The ability of agmatine to stimulate release of luteinizing hormone-releasing hormone has only been demonstrated *in vitro* i.e. by adding agmatine to cultured cells extracted from rat brains (2).

The ability of agmatine to stimulate human growth hormone release has not been demonstrated in animal or human studies. Human growth hormone releasing hormone which has been artificially modified to include agmatine as part of its structure (specifically at postion 29 of the amino acid sequence) has been shown *in vitro* to have greater GH-releasing potency in animal studies (3).

The ability of agmatine to stimulate increased secretion of insulin from islet cells has only been demonstrated in an *in vitro* animal study on rats (4). However even if oral supplementation of agmatine increased insulin release in humans this would seem to contradict the supplements claimed benefit of improved body composition. While insulin does have an anabolic effect and will increase muscle growth, it also causes growth of adipocytes (fat cells) and so tends to make individuals fatter. Agents which truly promote improved body composition do not cause increased secretion of insulin but rather improve the sensitivity of muscle cells to the effects of insulin. This allows the muscle cells to uptake more nutrients from the bloodstream and leaves less available to be taken up by adipocytes and stored in the form of fat.

In addition, animal studies indicate that agmatine may have a separate insulin-like effect on adipocytes causing them to increase their rate of lipogenesis (increased rate of fat storage) (5), (6).

The claims of an analgesic action for agmatine have not been demonstrated. One study on rats did show that agmatine enhanced morphine analgesia, but had no effect when administered on its own (7). In any case since agmatine is not licensed for this use in humans there are perhaps safer alternatives for the relief of post-workout pain, such as an over the counter pain killer from the local pharmacy.

Commonly used dosages

Agmatine is usually included as part of a proprietary formulation in commercial sport supplement preparations with the exact quantity of the substance not listed in the ingredients.

It is not usually sold as a stand alone supplement.

Safety

No known safety issues.

Interactions

None known.

References

1. Raasch W, Regunathan S, Li G, Reis DJ. Agmatine, the bacterial amine, is widely distributed in mammalian tissues. Life Sci. 1995;56:2319–2330
2. Kalra SP, Pearson E, Sahu A, Kalra PS. Agmatine, a novel hypothalamic amine, stimulates pituitary luteinizing hormone release in vivo and hypothalamic luteinizing hormone-releasing hormone release in vitro. Neurosci Lett 1995;194:165-168
3. Zarandi M, Serfozo P, Zsigo J, Deutch AH, Janaky T, Olsen DB, Bajusz S, Schally AV. Potent agonists of growth hormone-releasing hormone. II. Pept Res. 1992;5(4):190-3.
4. Sener, A. Lebrun, P. Blachier, F. Malaisse, W J. Stimulus-secretion coupling of arginine-induced insulin release. Insulinotropic action of agmatine. Biochem. Pharmacol. 1989;38(2):327–330

5. Pfeiffer B, Sarrazin W, Weitzel G. Insulin-like effects of agmatine derivatives in vitro and in vivo (author's transl). Hoppe Seylers Z Physiol Chem. 1981;362(10):1331-7.
6. Weitzel G, Pfeiffer B, Stock W. Insulin-like partial effects of agmatine derivatives in adipocytes. Hoppe Seylers Z Physiol Chem. 1980;361(1):51-60
7. Kolesnikov Y, Jain S, Pasternak GW. Modulation of opioid analgesia by agmatine. Eur J Pharmacol. 1996;296:17-22

Allothiamine

Other names

None

Star rating

1

What is it?

The word allothiamine does not appear in any chemical, phytochemical, herbal or medicinal database. However the word allo-thiamine suggests it is a form of the vitamin thiamine (the prefix allo signifies "form" or "isomer"). Thiamine is a water-soluble B vitamin, also known as vitamin B_1 which is involved in many metabolic processes in the human body including the conversion of carbohydrates into energy and supporting the function of heart, muscles and nervous system (1).

Allothiamine may be a form of allithiamine which is a lipophilic form of thiamine with better bioavailability. Allithiamine was isolated from garlic (Allium sativum) extracts in 1951 and it was later shown that allicin, an active principle of garlic which gives it its characteristic odour, conjugates with thiamine to form allithiamine which has the formula 2'-methyl-4'-amino-pyrimidyl-(5-methylformamino-5-hydroxy-2-pentenyl-(3)-allyl disulfide (2).

Claimed benefits

"A powerful neural stimulant that will increase concentration and focus during your workout." (3)

Mode of Action

No data found.

Effectiveness

No known data showing effectiveness.

Commonly used dosages

Allothiamine is included as part of a proprietary formulation in a commercial sport supplement preparation with the exact quantity of the substance not listed in the ingredients.

It is not sold as a stand alone supplement.

Safety

No known safety issues.

Interactions

None known.

References

1. MedlinePlus [online] at
    http://www.nlm.nih.gov/medlineplus/ency/article/002
    401.htm
2. Lonsdale D, Allithiamine and its Synthetic Derivatives: a
    Review. J Nutr Environ Med 1991;2:305-311
3. Gaspari Nutrition, Frequently Asked Questions [online]
    at http://store.gasparinutrition.com/product-
    faqs/2.html

Alpha Glycerylphosphorycholine

Other names

Alpha Glycerol Phosphoryl Choline
Alpha-GPC
Choline Alfoscerate
Glycero-3-Phosphocholine.
Glycerophosphocholine
L-alpha-Glycerophosphocholine
L-alpha-Glycerophosphorylcholine
SN-glycero-3-phosphocholine

Star rating

1

What is it?

"A component of PHOSPHATIDYLCHOLINES (lecithins), in which the two hydroxy groups of GLYCEROL are esterified with fatty acids. (From Stedman, 26th ed) It counteracts the effects of urea on enzymes and other macromolecules." (1)

Claimed benefits

Improves concentration, focus and memory. May also increase levels of growth hormone.

Mode of Action

Following administration alpha glycerylphosphorycholine is broken down by the enzyme glycerolphosphorylcholine diesterase to form glycerophosphate and choline (2).

Choline is an essential nutrient in humans, which although it can be synthesized by the body, this does not occur in sufficient quantities to meet the body's metabolic needs. Hence the majority of the body's choline must be ingested from the diet.

Choline is necessary for the synthesis of the neurotransmitter acetylcholine which is involved in muscle control and memory. Alpha glycerylphosphorycholine is thought to work by increasing levels of choline and therefore increasing the synthesis of acetylcholine.

Effectiveness

There is no known evidence that alpha glycerylphosphorycholine improves focus and concentration in a manner which improves sporting performance.

There is some evidence that administration of alpha glycerylphosphorycholine can improve memory and cognitive performance in people suffering from Alzheimers's disease (3), people recovering from cerebral ischemic attacks (stroke) (4) and in people suffering from vascular dementia (5). It has also been seen to prevent the impairment of attention and memory induced by the drug scopolamine in healthy individuals (6). However more research is needed to confirm whether attention and memory of normal healthy individuals can be improved by supplementation with alpha glycerylphosphorycholine.

The ability of alpha glycerylphosphorycholine to increase the release of human growth hormone has only been demonstrated in humans when it is administered together with Growth Hormone Releasing Hormone (7). Its ability to affect levels when administered alone has not been tested.

Commonly used dosages

Alpha glycerylphosphorycholine is usually included as part of a proprietary formulation in commercial sport supplement preparations with the exact quantity of the substance not listed in the ingredients. When the quantity is listed an amount of 50-100mg is common.

In the studies mentioned above where alpha glycerylphosphorycholine showed memory and cognition improvements in patients suffering from Alzheimer's, cerebral ischemia and vascular dementia a dose of 1200mg per day was used.

Safety

No known safety issues.

Interactions

May reduce the effectiveness of scopolamine (6).

References

1. Medical Dictionary Online [online] at http://www.online-medical-dictionary.org/L-alpha-Glycerylphosphorylcholine.asp?q=L-alpha-Glycerylphosphorylcholine
2. Gatti G, Barzaghi N, Acuto G, et al. A comparative study of free plasma choline levels following intramuscular administration of L alphaglycerylphosphorylcholine and citocholine in normal volunteers. Int J Clin Pharmacol Ther Toxicol 1992;30:331-5.
3. Moreno MDM. Cognitive improvement in mild to moderate Alzheimer's dementia after treatment with the acetylcholine precursor choline alfoscerate: A multicenter, double-blind, randomized, placebo-controlled trial. Clin Ther 2003;25:178-93
4. Barbagallo Sangiorgi G, Barbagallo M, Giordano M, *et al.* Alphaglycerophosphocholine in the mental recovery of cerebral ischemic attacks: An Italian multicenter clinical trial. Ann N Y Acad Sci 1994;717:253-69.
5. Di Perri R, Coppola G, Ambrosio LA, *et al.* A multicentre trial to the evaluate the efficacy and tolerability of alpha-glycerylphosphorylcholine versus cytosine diphosphocholine in patients with vascular dementia. J Int Med Res 1991;19:330-41.
6. Canal N, Franceschi M, Alberoni M, *et al.* Effect of L-alpha glycerylphosphorylcholine on amnesia caused by scopolamine. Int J Clin Pharmacol Ther Toxicol 1991;29:103-7.
7. Ceda GP, Ceresini G, Denti L, Marzani G, Piovani E, Banchini A, Tarditi E, Valenti G. alpha-Glycerylphosphorylcholine administration increases the

GH responses to GHRH of young and elderly subjects. Horm Metab Res. 1992;24(3):119-21.

Alpha-Ketoglutarate

Other names

2-ketoglutarate
2-ketoglutaric acid
2-Oxoglutamate
2-oxoglutarate
2-oxoglutarate(2-)
2-oxoglutaric acid
2-oxopentanedioate
Alpha-ketoglutarate
Alpha-ketoglutaric acid
Calcium Alpha-Ketoglutarate
Oxoglutaric acid

Star rating

3

What is it?

The carbon skeleton of glutamine.

Claimed benefits

Increases serum levels of amino acids, improves amino acid metabolism and promotes protein synthesis.

Mode of Action

The effect of supplemental alpha-ketoglutarate is to spare the amino acids histidine, proline and arginine from being transaminated in the TCA (tricarbonic acid) cycle to produce glutamate and hence increasing plasma levels of these amino acids.

It also increases serum levels of alpha-ketoisocaproate which is the alpha-ketoanalog of leucine. Alpha-ketoisocaproate acts an activator of protein synthesis (1).

Effectiveness

The above mentioned effects have been observed in tests on patients with chronic renal failure undergoing hemodialysis (1) and in tests on patients recovering from hip replacement operations (2).

In the tests involving hemodialysis patients maximal effects were observed after one year of supplementation. Interestingly after six months, plasma levels of histidine and proline (but not the other amino acids tested) were actually higher than the healthy control subjects. The other amino acids tested all rose but remained lower than healthy controls even at the one year mark.

In tests on patients recovering from hip replacement operations administration of alpha-ketoglutarate prevented the post-operative reduction in free muscle glutamine and protein synthesis which was observed in the non-supplemented patients.

There is some evidence from a small trial of six healthy males (3) that alpha-ketoglutarate can produce similar effects in healthy people however more work is needed to assess the level of these effects and whether or not they can produce any significant improvement in athletic performance in either the short or long term.

Commonly used dosages

Alpha-ketoglutarate is usually included as part of a proprietary formulation in commercial sport supplement preparations with the exact quantity of the substance not listed in the ingredients.

It is not usually sold as a stand alone supplement. It is commonly combined with either arginine or ornithine and sold as arginine alpha-ketoglutarate (AAKG) or ornithine alpha-ketoglutarate (OAKG).

In the studies mentioned above doses of approximately 3g per day were used.

Safety

No known safety issues.

Interactions

None known.

References

1. Riedel E, Nundel M, Hampl H. Alpha-Ketoglutarate application in hemodialysis patients improves amino acid metabolism. Nephron 1996;74:261-5.
2. Blomqvist BI, Hammarqvist F, von der Decken A, Wernerman J. Glutamine and alpha-ketoglutarate prevent the decrease in muscle free glutamine

concentration and influence protein synthesis after total hip replacement. Metabolism. 1995;44(9):1215-22

3. Cynober L, Coudray-Lucas C, de Bandt JP, Guéchot J, Aussel C, Salvucci M *et al.* Action of ornithine alpha-ketoglutarate, ornithine hydrochloride, and calcium alpha-ketoglutarate on plasma amino acid and hormonal patterns in healthy subjects. J Am Coll Nutr. 1990;9(1):2-12

Arachidonic Acid

Other names

5,8,11,14-Eicosatetraenoic acid
Eicosanetetraenoic acid
Icosa-5,8,11,14-tetraenoic acid

Star rating

1

What is it?

An unsaturated essential fatty acid used in the body as a precursor in the formation of prostaglandins, thromboxanes, and leukotrienes. It is synthesized from linoleic acid, an omega-6 fatty acid which is found mainly in vegetable oils, nuts and seeds.

Claimed benefits

Increased muscle growth.

Mode of Action

Arachidonic acid is present in the phospholipids which form cell membranes. Exercise causes the enzyme phospholipase A2 to release arachidonic acid into the cell cytoplasm where it is converted by the enzyme cyclooxygenase-2 (COX-2) into prostaglandins. These prostaglandins bind to receptors within the cell and initiate signalling cascades which lead to muscle growth (1), (2).

Effectiveness

There is no evidence that supplementation with arachidonic acid causes increased muscle growth.

In a small study funded by a supplement manufacturer (3) arachidonic acid supplementation of 1000mg/day did not yield statistically significant changes in body mass or composition.

Commonly used dosages

1000mg/day

Safety

Various studies have shown no adverse effects in doses up to 1500mg/day (4).

Interactions

None known.

References

1. Rao, G. N., N. R. Madamanchi, M. Lele, L. Gadiparthi, A. C. Gingras, T. E. Eling, and N. Sonenberg. A potential role for extracellular signal-regulated kinases in prostaglandin F2alpha-induced protein synthesis in smooth muscle cells. J Biol Chem. 1999;274:12925-12932.
2. Trappe, T. A., F. White, C. P. Lambert, D. Cesar, M. Hellerstein, and W. J. Evans. Effect of ibuprofen and acetaminophen on postexercise muscle protein synthesis. Am J Physiol Endocrinol Metab. 2002;282:E551-556.
3. Roberts MD, Iosia M, Kerksick CM, Taylor LW, Campbell B *et al*. Effects of arachidonic acid supplementation on training adaptations in resistance-trained males. J Int Soc Sports Nutr. 2007;4:21
4. Calder PC. Dietary arachidonic acid: harmful, harmless or helpful? British Journal of Nutrition 2007;98:451–453

Avena Sativa

Other names

A. byzantina
A. diffusa
Avena Fructus
Avenae herba
Avenae stramentum
Oat

Star rating

1

What is it?

A cereal grain commonly used as food.

Claimed benefits

Increased levels of testosterone.

Mode of Action

97% of circulating testosterone is bound to circulating proteins produced in the liver. Most is bound to sex hormone binding globulin (SHBG) and a smaller amount is also bound to a protein called albumin. Only the 3% which is unbound (free testosterone) is available to act on tissues (1).

It is variously claimed that plant saponins derived from oat called avenacosides A & B can either release testosterone from SHBG or reduce levels of SHBG so that less is available to bind testosterone.

Others claim that avenacosides A & B can stimulate the pituitary to release more luteinizing hormone which in turn stimulates the testes to produce more testosterone.

Effectiveness

No evidence exists that avenacosides A & B have any effect on SHBG.

A study published in a Japanese journal in 1976 (2) claimed that avenacosides A & B can cause release of luteinizing hormone. However it only showed an effect in rats, not humans. This result has never been confirmed or replicated in any subsequent studies.

Commonly used dosages

For the purposes of cholesterol reduction (which IS a proven benefit of oat consumption) 50 - 150 grams of oat equivalent to between 3 and 10 grams of beta-glucan (the soluble fibre component of oat) are usually recommended (3).

In sports supplements avena sativa is commonly included in amounts between 50 mg and 500 mg usually as part of a proprietary blend of various ingredients.

Safety

No known safety issues.

Interactions

None known.

References

1. Marshall WJ, Bangert SK. Clinical Chemistry 5th Edition. Philadelphia, Elsevier Ltd; 2004
2. Fukushima M, Watanabe S, Kushima K. Extraction and purification of a substance with luteinizing hormone releasing activity from the leaves of Avena Sativa. Tohoku J Exp Med. 1976;119(2):115-122.
3. Braaten JT, Wood PJ, Scott FW. *et al.* Oat beta-glucan reduces blood cholesterol concentration in hypercholesterolemic subjects. Eur J Clin Nutr 1994;48:465-74.

Bacopa Monniera

Other names

Bacopa Monnieri
Brahmi
Herpestis monniera
Indian Pennywort
Jalanimba
Moniera cuneifolia
Thyme-Leave Gratiola
Waterhyssop

Star rating

2

What is it?

A herb of the Scrophulariaceae family traditionally used in Indian Ayurvedic medicine.

Claimed benefits

Improved memory and cognitive stimulant.
Fat loss and cortisol suppression.

Mode of Action

The active component is thought to be steroidal saponins present in the leaves, in particular bacosides A & B (1). The exact mode of action of these compounds in the brain is unknown but is probably via a combination of;

- acetylcholine release
- choline acetylase activity

- muscarinic cholinergic receptor binding, and
- anti-oxidant action (2).

The fat loss effects are claimed to be due to a cortisol suppressing action since cortisol is involved in body fat accumulation especially abdominal fat.

Effectiveness

There is some evidence from animal (3) and human experiments (2), (4) that Bacopa Monniera improves learning and memory in healthy subjects. However there is no known data showing that this has a beneficial effect on sporting performance.

Bacopa Monniera has been shown in one study on rats to reduce blood levels of corticosterone (another hormone similar to cortisol which is also released in response to stress) when the rats were subjected to stress (5).

In other studies Bacopa Monniera appears to improve depression in animals (6) (7) and humans (8). Cortisol is sometimes raised in humans with depression however cortisol levels were not tested in these studies.

Unfortunately there is no other evidence that Bacopa Monniera can reduce cortisol levels in healthy humans or that it has any effects on body fat.

Commonly used dosages

Bacopa Monniera is usually included as part of a proprietary formulation in commercial sport supplement preparations with the exact quantity of the substance not listed in the ingredients. When the quantity is listed an amount of 50-100mg is common.

When sold as a stand alone supplement capsules of 100 to 250mg are commonly seen with a recommended dose of one to three capsules per day.

In the human studies cited above showing improvements in memory, participants took 300mg per day of an extract standardized for bacosides A and B (no less than 55% of combined bacosides).

Safety

No known safety issues.

Interactions

None known.

References

1. Kidd PM. A review of nutrients and botanicals in the integrative management of cognitive dysfunction. Altern Med Rev 1999;4:144-61.
2. Stough C, Lloyd J, Clarke J, et al. The chronic effects of an extract of Bacopa monniera (Brahmi) on cognitive function in healthy human subjects. Psychopharmacology 2001;156:481-4.
3. Singh HK, Dhawan BN. Neuropsychopharmacological effects of the Ayurvedic nootropic Bacopa monniera Linn. (Brahmi). Indian J Pharmacol 1997:29(5); 359-365
4. Roodenrys S, Booth D, Bulzomi S, Phipps A, Micallef C, Smoker J. Chronic Effects of Brahmi (Bacopa monnieri) on Human Memory. Neuropsychopharmacology 2002;27:279–281
5. Sheikh N, Ahmad A, Siripurapu KB, Kuchibhotla VK, Singh S, Palit G. Effect of Bacopa monniera on stress induced changes in plasma corticosterone and brain

monoamines in rats. J Ethnopharmacol 2007;111(3):671-676
6. Zhou Y, Shen YH, Zhang C, Su J, Liu RH, Zhang WD. Triterpene Saponins from Bacopa monnieri and Their Antidepressant Effects in Two Mice Models. J. Nat. Prod 2007;70(4):652–655
7. Sairam K, Dorababu M, Goel RK, Bhattacharya SK. Antidepressant activity of standardized extract of Bacopa monniera in experimental models of depression in rats. Phytomedicine. 2002;9(3):207-11
8. Calabrese C, Gregory WL, Leo M, Kraemer D, Bone K, Oken B. Effects of a Standardized Bacopa monnieri Extract on Cognitive Performance, Anxiety, and Depression in the Elderly: A Randomized, Double-Blind, Placebo-Controlled Trial. J Altern Complement Med 2008;14(6):707-713

Banaba

Other names

Crepe Myrtle
Lagerstroemia speciosa
Pride of India
Queens Crape Myrtle
Queen's Flower

Star rating

3

What is it?

A tropical deciduous flowering tree. The leaves of Banaba are used in traditional medicine in the Phillipines as a treatment for diabetes.

Claimed benefits

Weight loss and improvement in body composition (less fat tissue and more lean muscle mass).

Mode of Action

Several compounds have been isolated from the leaves of Banaba which can lower blood glucose levels, activate insulin receptors, improve cellular sensitivity to insulin and prevent weight gain.

Effectiveness

Three active ellagitannins, lagerstroemin, flosin B and reginin A have been identified as present in Banaba leaves and shown *in vitro* to enhance glucose transport and increase glucose uptake of rat adipocytes (1). In addition lagerstroemin has been demonstrated *in vitro* to activate insulin receptors in rat adipocytes and in hamster cells modified to express human insulin receptors. The proposed mechanism of action is that lagerstroemin binds to the insulin receptor in a different location to insulin (2).

In vivo studies in non insulin dependent diabetic mice have shown the ability of Banaba extract (not standardized for any particular component) to reduce blood glucose levels (3) and prevent increases in body weight and fat tissue (4).

In the only human study conducted with Banaba, ten Type II non insulin dependent diabetics received an extract of Banaba standardized to contain 1% corosolic acid in doses ranging from 16mg to 48mg. A statistically significant drop in blood glucose levels was seen at the 48mg dose (5).

Further studies are required to confirm whether Banaba can have similar effects in healthy individuals.

Commonly used dosages

Banaba is often included as part of a proprietary formulation in commercial sport supplement preparations with the exact quantity of the substance not listed in the ingredients. When the quantity is listed an amount of 50mg is common.

It is not usually sold as a stand alone supplement.

In the study cited above where an effect on blood glucose levels was demonstrated in diabetic humans a dose of 48mg was used, (standardized to contain 1% corosolic acid).

Safety

No known safety issues.

Interactions

May increase the blood glucose lowering effect of diabetes medications.

References

1. Hayashi T, Maruyama H, Kasai R, Hattori K, Takasuga S, Hazeki O *et al*. Ellagitannins from Lagerstroemia speciosa as activators of glucose transport in fat cells. Planta Med 2002;68:173-5.

2. Hattori K, Sukenobu N, Sasaki T, Takasuga S, Hayashi T, Kasai R *et al.* Activation of insulin receptors by lagerstroemin. J Pharmacol Sci 2003;93:69-73.
3. Kakuda T, Sakane I, Takihara T, Ozaki Y, Takeuchi H, Kuroyanagi M. Hypoglycemic effect of extracts from Lagerstroemia speciosa L. leaves in genetically diabetic KK-AY mice. Biosci Biotechnol Biochem 1996;60:204-8.
4. Suzuki Y, Unno T, Ushitani M, Hayashi K, Kakuda T. Antiobesity activity of extracts from Lagerstroemia speciosa L. leaves on female KK-Ay mice. J Nutr Sci Vitaminol (Tokyo) 1999;45:791-5.
5. Judy WV, Hari SP, Stogsdill WW, Judy JS, Naguib YM, Passwater R. Antidiabetic activity of a standardized extract (Glucosol) from Lagerstroemia speciosa leaves in Type II diabetics. A dose-dependence study. J Ethnopharmacol 2003;87:115-7.

BCAAs

Other names

Branched chain amino acids

Star rating

4

What is it?

The essential amino acids L-leucine, L-isoleucine and L-valine. In common with most amino acids BCAAs can be used for protein synthesis but unlike other amino acids can also be used directly by muscles for energy without requiring prior gluconeogenesis in the liver.

There are no official recommended daily intakes for BCAAs and average daily requirements for adult males have been calculated as being anywhere from 44mg/kg per day to 144mg/kg per day (1).

Claimed benefits

Increases lean muscle mass, improves recovery from exercise and reduces post exercise muscle soreness.

Mode of Action

BCAAs particularly leucine, exert anabolic effects by increasing the rate of muscle protein synthesis and decreasing the rate of muscle protein breakdown (2).

They seem to achieve this by increasing signalling in the muscle cell mTOR pathway which increases protein synthesis (3) and by increasing the sensitivity of muscle protein synthesis to the anabolic action of insulin (4) (5).

Effectiveness

The ability of BCAA to improve recovery and reduce post exercise muscle soreness and fatigue has been seen in several studies. For example when 5g of BCAAs (in a leucine:isoleucine:valine ratio 2.3:1:1.2) was given to men and women 15 minutes before performing 7 sets of 20 squats the duration of muscle soreness and fatigue over the following days was reduced compared to placebo (6).

Similar reductions in muscle soreness and fatigue as well as reductions in blood markers of muscle damage were seen in long distance runners supplemented with a BCAA drink during training (7). Reduced muscle soreness has also been seen in weight trainers (8) and measures of amino acid metabolism in cyclists given BCAAs showed a protein-sparing effect during recovery after exercise (9).

In terms of effects on muscle mass, a placebo controlled double blind study of 16 subjects undertaking a 21 day high altitude trek examined the effects of supplementation with BCAAs (5.76, 2.88 and 2.88 g per day of leucine, isoleucine and valine). After altitude exposure both groups showed a loss of body mass but the BCAA group showed increased lean mass of 1.5%, as opposed to no change in the placebo group. Arm muscle cross-sectional area also tended to increase in the BCAA group, whereas there was a significant decrease of 6.8% in placebo. These results suggest that the BCAA group had been synthesizing muscle tissue while the placebo group had been catabolizing (10).

In another study 10 weight training males given 14g/day of BCAAs (leucine:isoleucine:valine ratio 2:1:1) for 30 days showed significant increases in fat free mass averaging 0.8kg (11).

Commonly used dosages

A wide variety of daily dosages of BCAAs seem to be recommended from 5g/day up to 20g/day.

BCAAs are sold with a variety of leucine, isoleucine, valine ratios although the ratio most frequently sold is 2:1:1. Some manufacturers provide other ratios based on varying claims such as the ratio mimicking the ratio of BCAAs found in muscle.

There is little agreement among official sources as to the optimal dietary ratio or total amount necessary of BCAAs. The 2:1:1 ratio commonly quoted seems to be supported by the majority of the studies (1) and is roughly equivalent to the ratio of BCAAs recommended by the USA National Institutes of Health in its Dietary Reference Intakes (DRI) for protein intake which recommends a ratio of 2:0.9:1.7 (12).

Although the scientific literature records that BCAAs make up 14–18% of the total amino acids in muscle proteins I have not been able to find any research which records the proportion of the individual BCAAs in human muscle. Figures are recorded for rat muscle which has a protein bound leucine:isoleucine:valine ratio of approximately 2:1:1 (13).

Safety

While high doses of BCAAs have been reported to cause nausea amounts as high as 60g/day have been used safely for short periods of 7 days (14).

Interactions

Amino acids can stimulate insulin release so there is a possibility BCAAs may increase the hypoglycemic effect of diabetic medication (15).

BCAAs may increase the risk of liver toxicity in patients taking sodium valproate. People on this medication should avoid BCAAs (14).

References

1. Riazi R, Wykes LJ, Ball RO, Pencharz PB. The total branched-chain amino acid requirement in young healthy adult men determined by indicator amino acid oxidation by use of L-[1-13C]phenylalanine. J Nutr. 2003;133(5):1383-9

2. Blomstrand E, Eliasson J, Karlsson HK, Köhnke R. Branched-chain amino acids activate key enzymes in protein synthesis after physical exercise. J Nutr. 2006;136(1 Suppl):269S-73S

3. Rennie MJ, Bohé J, Smith K, Wackerhage H, Greenhaff P. Branched-chain amino acids as fuels and anabolic signals in human muscle. J Nutr. 2006;136(1 Suppl):264S-8S

4. Garlick PJ, Grant I. Amino acid infusion increases the sensitivity of muscle protein synthesis in vivo to insulin. Effect of branched-chain amino acids. Biochem J. 1988;254(2):579-84

5. Garlick PJ. The role of leucine in the regulation of protein metabolism. J Nutr. 2005;135(6 Suppl):1553S-6S

6. Shimomura Y, Yamamoto Y, Bajotto G, Sato J, Murakami T *et al.* Nutraceutical effects of branched-chain amino acids on skeletal muscle. J Nutr. 2006;136(2):529S-532S

7. Matsumoto K, Koba T, Hamada K, Sakurai M, Higuchi T, Miyata H. Branched-chain amino acid supplementation attenuates muscle soreness, muscle damage and inflammation during an intensive training program. J Sports Med Phys Fitness. 2009;49(4):424-31

8. Jackman SR, Witard OC, Jeukendrup AE, Tipton KD. Branched-chain amino acid ingestion can ameliorate soreness from eccentric exercise. Med Sci Sports Exerc. 2010;42(5):962-70

9. Blomstrand E, Saltin B. BCAA intake affects protein metabolism in muscle after but not during exercise in humans. Am J Physiol Endocrinol Metab. 2001;281(2):E365-74

10. Schena F, Guerrini F, Tregnaghi P, Kayser B. Branched-chain amino acid supplementation during trekking at high altitude. The effects on loss of body mass, body composition, and muscle power. Eur J Appl Physiol Occup Physiol. 1992;65(5):394-8

11. Candeloro N, Bertini I, Melchiorri G, De Lorenzo A. [Effects of prolonged administration of branched-chain amino acids on body composition and physical fitness]. [Article in Italian] Minerva Endocrinol. 1995;20(4):217-23
12. National Institutes of Health. Office of Dietary Supplements. Nutrient Recommendations. [online] at http://ods.od.nih.gov/Health_Information/Dietary_Ref erence_Intakes.aspx
13. The National Academies Press. Dietary Reference Intakes for Energy, Carbohydrate, Fiber, Fat, Fatty Acids, Cholesterol, Protein, and Amino Acids (Macronutrients) (2005) (page 597) [online] at http://books.nap.edu/openbook.php?record_id=10490 &page=597
14. Scarna A, Gijsman HJ, McTavish SF, Harmer CJ, Cowen PJ, Goodwin GM. Effects of a branched-chain amino acid drink in mania. Br J Psychiatry. 2003;182:210-3
15. van Loon LJ, Kruijshoop M, Menheere PP, Wagenmakers AJ, Saris WH, Keizer HA. Amino acid ingestion strongly enhances insulin secretion in patients with long-term type 2 diabetes. Diabetes Care. 2003;26(3):625-30

Benfotiamine

Other names

Benphothiamine
Benzenecarbothioic acid S-[2-[[(4-amino-2-methyl-5-pyrimidinyl)methyl] formylamino]-1-[2-(phosphonooxy)ethyl]-1-propenyl] ester
Betivina
Biotamin
Nitanevril

S-[(Z)-2-[(4-amino-2-methylpyrimidin-5-yl)methyl-
formylamino]-5- phosphonooxypent-2-en-3-yl]
benzenecarbothioate
S-benzoylthiamine O-monophosphate
Thiobenzoic acid S-ester with N-[(4-amino-2-methyl-5-
pyrimidinyl)methyl]-N-(4-hydroxy-2-mercapto-1-methyl-1-
butenyl)formamide O-phosphate
Vitanevril

Star rating

1

What is it?

A synthetic amphiphilic S-acyl derivative of the vitamin
thiamine which has a higher bioavailability than thiamine.

Claimed benefits

Reduces cellular damage caused by Advanced Glycation End-
products (AGE's).
Promotes healthy nerve function.
Enhances blood sugar utilization and increases energy
production.

Note: AGE's are a group of sugar derived molecules such as
N-carboxymethyl-lysine, pentosidine, or methylglyoxal
derivatives which are the end result of a series of biochemical
processes which glucose undergoes in the body. In normal
individuals AGE's are formed at a slow constant rate,
however in diabetics the increased availability of glucose
causes them to form and accumulate at an accelerated rate.
AGE's react with cellular proteins altering their structure and
it is believed that they are the cause of almost all of the
pathological complications of diabetes (1).

Mode of Action

It is believed that benfotiamine activates the pentose phosphate enzyme transketolase which removes compounds (probably glyceraldehyde 3-phosphate and fructose 6-phosphate) which are necessary components in the biochemical pathway for the production of AGE's (2).

Effectiveness

There is some evidence that benfotiamine is beneficial for the prevention of diabetic complications (1), (3), (4), (5). However there is no evidence that it produces any improvement in sporting performance in normal individuals beyond promoting general health by adequate intake of the vitamin thiamine. There is no evidence that it enhances energy production or improves nerve function.

Commonly used dosages

Benfotiamine is usually included as part of a proprietary formulation in commercial sport supplement preparations with the exact quantity of the substance not listed in the ingredients. When the quantity is listed an amount of 50mg is typical.

When sold as a stand alone supplement capsules or tablets of 50 – 150mg are common.

In the studies examining the effects of benfotiamine supplementation in diabetics doses of 1000mg/day were used.

Safety

No known safety issues.

Interactions

None known.

References

1. Peppa M, Uribarri J, Vlassara H. Glucose, Advanced Glycation End Products, and Diabetes Complications: What Is New and What Works. Clinical Diabetes 2003;21:186-187
2. Volvert M, Seyen S, Piette M, Evrard B, Gangolf M, Plumier J, *et al*. Benfotiamine, a synthetic S-acyl thiamine derivative, has different mechanisms of action and a different pharmacological profile than lipid-soluble thiamine disulfide derivatives. BMC Pharmacol 2008;8:10
3. Stirban A, Negrean M, Stratmann B, Götting C, Salomon J, Kleesiek K, *et al*. Adiponectin decreases postprandially following a heat-processed meal in individuals with type 2 diabetes: an effect prevented by benfotiamine and cooking method. Diabetes Care 2007;30(10):2514-6
4. Stirban A, Negrean M, Stratmann B, Gawlowski T, Horstmann T, Götting C, *et al*. Benfotiamine prevents macro- and microvascular endothelial dysfunction and oxidative stress following a meal rich in advanced glycation end products in individuals with type 2 diabetes. Diabetes Care 2006;29(9):2064-71
5. Babaei-Jadidi R, Karachalias N, Ahmed N, Battah S, Thornalley PJ. Prevention of incipient diabetic nephropathy by high-dose thiamine and benfotiamine. Diabetes. 2003;52(8):2110-20

Berberine

Other names

5,6-Dihydro-9,10-dimethoxybenzo[g]-1,3-benzodioxolo[5,6-a]quinolizinium
7,8,13,13a-tetradehydro-9,10-dimethoxy-2,3-(methylenedioxy)berbinium
9,10-Dimethoxy-2,3-(methylenedioxy)-7,8,13,13a-tetrahydroberbinium
Berberine sulfate
Umbellatine

Star rating

4

What is it?

A plant alkaloid present in over nine botanical families but mainly in the Berberidaceae family (1) which includes berberis species, also known as barberry. It is also found in goldenseal (Hydrastis canadensis) and coptis or goldenthread (Coptis chinensis). It is used in traditional Chinese and Ayurvedic medicine for a variety of ailments including heart failure, burns and infections.

Claimed benefits

Weight loss and improvement in body composition (less fat tissue and more lean muscle mass.

Mode of Action

Improved cellular insulin sensitivity and lowering of blood glucose levels.

Effectiveness

The ability of berberine to increase cellular insulin sensitivity and promote weight loss has been demonstrated in animal models both *in vitro* (2), (3) and *in vivo* (4), (5), (6). Berberine was also seen to downregulate the expression of genes involved in lipogenesis and upregulate those involved in energy expenditure in adipose tissue and muscle (4) and its *in vitro* glucose lowering ability was seen to be similar to the diabetes drug metformin (3).

In human studies with Type II non insulin dependent diabetics the glucose lowering effect of berberine was likewise found to be similar to metformin (7). In another randomized, double-blind, and placebo-controlled 4-clinical centre study of 116 patients carried out in China, also with Type II non insulin dependent diabetics, the glucose lowering ability of berberine was confirmed and found to be safe. It was also demonstrated to have a cholesterol lowering effect (8), (9).

Commonly used dosages

Berberine is often included as part of a proprietary formulation in commercial sport supplement preparations with the exact quantity of the substance not listed in the ingredients.

It is not usually sold as a stand alone supplement.

In the clinical trial cited above where an effect on blood glucose levels was demonstrated in diabetic humans a dose of 1000mg per day was used.

5

Safety

Should not be used in pregnancy or by infants as there is a risk to the fetus and newborn infants of developing kernicterus (10).

Interactions

Berberine interacts with cyclosporine by increasing the levels in the blood of this drug. They should not be taken together (11).

References

1. The Merck Index 14th Ed. New Jersey, Merck & Co. Inc. 2006.
2. Ko B, Choi SB, Park SK, Jang JS, Kim YE, Park S. Insulin Sensitizing and Insulinotropic Action of Berberine from Cortidis Rhizoma. Biol Pharm Bull 2005;28(8):1431
3. Yin J, Hu R, Chen M, Tang J, Li F, Yang Y, Chen J. Effects of berberine on glucose metabolism in vitro. Metabolism 2002;51(11): 1439-1443
4. Lee YS, Kim WS, Kim KH, Yoon MJ, Cho HJ, Shen Y *et al.* Berberine, a Natural Plant Product, Activates AMP-Activated Protein Kinase With Beneficial Metabolic Effects in Diabetic and Insulin-Resistant States. Diabetes 2005;55:2256–2264
5. Yin J, Gao Z, Liu D, Liu Z, Ye J. Berberine improves glucose metabolism through induction of glycolysis. Am J Physiol Endocrinol Metab. 2008;294(1):E148-56.
6. Tang L, Wei W, Chen LM, Liu S. Effects of berberine on diabetes induced by alloxan and a high-fat/high-cholesterol diet in rats. J Ethnopharmacol 2006;108(1):109-115
7. Yin J, Xing H, Ye J. Efficacy of berberine in patients with type 2 diabetes mellitus. Metabolism. 2008;57(5):712-7.

8. Zhang Y, Li X, Zou D, Liu W, Yang J, Zhu N *et al.* Treatment of Type 2 Diabetes and Dyslipidemia with the Natural Plant Alkaloid Berberine. J Clin Endocrinol Metab 2008;93(7): 2559-2565
9. Clinicaltrials.gov [online] at http://clinicaltrials.gov/ct2/show/NCT00462046
10. Chan E. Displacement of bilirubin from albumin by berberine. Biol Neonate 1993;63:201-8.
11. Wu X, Li Q, Xin H, Yu A, Zhong M. Effects of berberine on the blood concentration of cyclosporin A in renal transplanted recipients: clinical and pharmacokinetic study. Eur J Clin Pharmacol 2005;61:567-72.

Bergenin

Other names

(2R,3S,4S,4aR,10bS)-3,4,8,10-tetrahydroxy-2-(hydroxymethyl)-9-methoxy-3,
4,4a,10b-tetrahydro-2H-pyrano[3,2-c]isochromen-6-one
3,4,8,10-tetrahydroxy-2-(hydroxymethyl)-9-methoxy-3,4,4a,10b-tetrahydropyrano[3,2-c]isochromen-6(2H)-one
Corylopsin
Cuscutin
Peltophorin

Star rating

2

What is it?

An isocoumarin, a C-glucoside of 4-O-methyl gallic acid (1), isolated from various medicinal plants. These include

Bergenia crassifolia (Siberian Tea), Astilbe thunbergii (Ostrich Plume) and Ardisia japonica (Marlberry Bush) plants.

Claimed benefits

Aids fat loss.

Mode of Action

Opposes the lipogenic (fat storage) action of insulin, and enhances the lipolytic (fat breakdown) effects of norepinephirine by enhancing the binding of norepinephrine to phospholipids (2).

(Norepinephrine also known as noradrenaline is a hormone and neurotransmitter which can increase the heart rate, trigger the release of glucose from energy stores, and increase blood flow to skeletal muscle.)

Effectiveness

There is only a single report of bergenine having these effects in a 1998 *in vitro* study using rat cells (2).

Commonly used dosages

Bergenin is usually included as part of a proprietary formulation in commercial sport supplement preparations with the exact quantity of the substance not listed in the ingredients.

It is not usually sold as a stand alone supplement.

Safety

No known safety issues.

Interactions

None known.

References

1. Ye YP, Sun HX, Pan YJ. Bergenin monohydrate from the rhizomae of Astilbe chinensis. Acta Cryst 2004;60:397-398
2. Han LK, Ninomiya H, Taniguchi M, Baba K, Kimura Y, Okuda H. Norepinephrine-augmenting lipolytic effectors from Astilbe thunbergii rhizomes. J Nat Prod. 1998;61(8):1006-11

Beta Alanine

Other names

2-Carboxyethylamine
3-Aminopropanoate
3-Aminopropanoic acid
3-Aminopropionic acid
3-Aminopropionsaeure
Abufene

Star rating

4

What is it?

A non essential amino acid which can be synthesized in the human body via dihydrouracil and carnosine pathways (1). Beta alanine is classed as a non-proteinogenic amino acid, as it is not used in the building of proteins (2).

Claimed benefits

Delays muscle fatigue, improves endurance, increases strength, increases lean muscle mass, improves body composition (more lean muscle tissue, less fat tissue).

Mode of Action

Beta alanine's effects are achieved indirectly through its ability to increase intra-muscular levels of carnosine.

Carnosine (β-alanyl-L-histidine) is a dipeptide synthesized from the precursors L-histidine and beta alanine by carnosine synthetase (3). It is present in high concentrations in skeletal muscle being more abundant in Type II (glycolytic) muscle fibres than Type I (oxidative) fibres (4), (5).

Intense exercise, particularly of the anaerobic type, results in the production of lactic acid in skeletal muscle which causes a drop in intramuscular pH i.e. it becomes more acidic and it is believed that this is one of the mechanisms which causes muscle fatigue and a reduction in power output (6).

Carnosine however is one of various physiological mechanisms which works to buffer this increase in acidity and maintain pH within its optimal physiological range (7) and hence delaying the onset of fatigue.

As mentioned previously, carnosine is composed of the amino acids histidine and beta alanine. Histidine is present in skeletal muscle in high concentrations (8), (9) whereas beta alanine is present in much lower concentrations and is therefore the rate limiting step in carnosine synthesis (10), (11), (12).

Oral supplementation with 6.4g of beta alanine daily has been shown to increase muscle carnosine concentrations in humans by approximately 60% at 4 weeks and approximately 80% at 10 weeks (12), (13).

Effectiveness

The ability of beta alanine to delay muscle fatigue and improve endurance has been demonstrated in at least three human studies.

After 4 weeks supplementation with 6.4g of beta alanine daily, the total work done before exhaustion in a cycling test performed by a group of 13 male subjects increased by 13% with a further 3% increase at 10 weeks compared to the placebo group (12).

In a study on 8 trained national level sprinters (and a placebo group of 7) supplementation with beta alanine for 4 weeks at 4.8g per day produced increases in torque of approximately 6% and 4% in sets 4 and 5 during 5 sets of knee extension exercises (3).

Finally a study performed on 11 women taking 6.4g of beta alanine for 28 days (with a placebo group also of 11) the beta alanine group showed an increase in physical working capacity at fatigue threshold of 13% and increase in the time to exhaustion of 2.5% in a cycling test (14).

It would be hoped as well as being logically surmised that these benefits could also lead to increases in strength, increases in lean muscle mass and improvements in body composition. As Kendrick *et al* (2) point out, the rationale being the ability of increased muscle carnosine to prolong each bout of resistance exercise (more repetitions per set) and in turn a greater mean volume of training per week. This increase in work resulting in an increase in mechanical stress and in turn a greater adaptive process occurring.

Unfortunately this has not materialized in any of the studies. That of Kendrick *et al* being perhaps the largest performed to date which looked specifically at the effects of 10 weeks of resistance training combined with beta alanine supplementation on whole body strength, force production, muscular endurance and body composition. Beta alanine was not found to improve any of these parameters (2).

Hoffman *et al* (15) comparing beta alanine with creatine plus beta alanine failed to find any differences in strength and power between the two groups. However they did report improvements in body composition in the beta alanine group but confusingly the results as they published them did not support this.

Similarly in the tests mentioned previously which showed the ability of beta alanine to delay muscle fatigue, in the first involving 13 males taking beta alanine for 10 weeks no effect on body mass was noted (12). In the second involving trained sprinters no improvement in 400 meter race time was seen (3) and finally in the cycling testing of 11 women there was no improvement in the maximal aerobic power generated (14).

In summary, beta alanine may be useful to those engaged in endurance sports but is unlikely to show much benefit to strength and power athletes. Perhaps the incremental work which it allows at the endurance threshold is simply too small to have an appreciable cumulative effect on muscle synthesis following resistance exercise.

Commonly used dosages

Beta alanine is available in a variety of capsules usually between 750mg –1000mg with recommended daily doses of between 2g and 6g.

It is also sold as a powder in tubs with similar daily recommended doses.

Beta alanine is also often included as part of a proprietary formulation in commercial sport supplement preparations with the exact quantity of the substance not listed in the ingredients.

Safety

No known safety issues. Beta alanine has been reported to cause a tingling or itching sensation in the skin lasting up to an hour after ingestion, but this is not known to be harmful.

Interactions

Beta alanine has been shown to reduce the absorption of the muscle relaxing drug baclofen in rats (16). It is not known if a similar effect occurs in humans but it may be wise to avoid taking them together.

References

1. Kegg Pathway Database [online] at
    http://www.genome.jp/dbget-
    bin/get_pathway?org_name=hsa&mapno=00410
2. Kendrick IP, Harris RC, Kim HJ, Kim CK, Dang VH,
    Thanh Q, *et al.* The effects of 10 weeks of resistance
    training combined with b-alanine supplementation on
    whole body strength, force production, muscular
    endurance and body composition. Amino Acids
    2008;34:547–554
3. Derave W, Ozdemir MS, Harris RC, Pottier A, Reyngoudt
    H, Koppo K *et al.* Beta alanine supplementation
    augments muscle carnosine content and attenuates
    fatigue during repeated isokinetic contraction bouts in
    trained sprinters. J Appl Physiol 2003;103:1736–1743
4. Dunnett M, Harris RC. High-performance liquid
    chromatographic determination of imidazole dipeptides,
    histidine, 1-methylhistidine and 3-methylhistidine in
    equine and camel muscle and individual muscle fibres. J
    Chromatogr B Biomed Appl 1997;688: 47–55
5. Harris RC, Dunnett M, Greenhaff PL. Carnosine and
    taurine contents in individual fibres of human vastus
    alteralis muscle. J Sports Sci 1998;16:639–643
6. Fitts RH, Holloszy JO. Lactate and contractile force in
    frog muscle during development of fatigue and recovery.
    Am J Physiol 1976;231: 430–409
7. Harris RC, Marlin DJ, Dunnett M, Snow DH, Hultman E.
    Muscle buffering capacity and dipeptide content in the
    thoroughbred horse, greyhound dog and man. Comp
    Biochem Physiol 1990;97A:249-251
8. Harris RC, Marlin DJ, Dunnett M, Snow DH, Hultman E.
    Muscle buffering capacity and dipeptide content in the
    thoroughbred horse, greyhound dog and man. Comp
    Biochem Physiol A 1990;97:249-51.

9. Horinishi H, Grillo M, Margolis FL. Purification and characterization of carnosine synthetase from mouse olfactory bulbs. J Neurochem 1978;31: 909–919

10. Bakardjiev A, Bauer K. Transport of beta-alanine and biosynthesis of carnosine by skeletal muscle cells in primary culture. Eur J Biochem 1994;225:617–623

11. Dunnett M, Harris RC. Influence of oral beta alanine and histidine supplementation on the carnosine content of the gluteus medius. Equine Vet J 1999;30, Suppl: 499–504

12. Hill CA, Harris RC, Kim HJ, Harris BD, Sale C, Boobis LH, *et al*. Influence of beta-alanine supplementation on skeletal muscle carnosine concentrations and high intensity cycling capacity. Amino Acids (Vienna) 2007;32: 225–233

13. Harris RC, Tallon MJ, Dunnett M, Boobis L, Coakley J, Kim HJ, *et al*. The absorption of orally supplied β-alanine and its effect on muscle carnosine synthesis in human vastus lateralis. Amino Acids 2006;30:279-89.

14. Stout JR, Cramer JT, Zoeller RF, Torok D, Costa P, Hoffman JR *et al*. Effects of beta-alanine supplementation on the onset of neuromuscular fatigue and ventilatory threshold in women. Amino Acids 2007;32:381-6.

15. Hoffman J, Raramess N, Kang J, Mangine G, Faigenbaum A, Stout J. Effect of creatine and beta-alanine supplementation on performance and endocrine responses in strength/power athletes. Int J Sport Nutr Exerc Metab 2006;16: 430-446

16. Polache A, Plá-Delfina JM, Merino M. Partially competitive inhibition of intestinal baclofen absorption by beta-alanine, a nonessential dietary aminoacid. Biopharm Drug Dispos. 1991;12(9):647-60

Beta Sitosterol

Other names

22:23-dihydrostigmasterol
24β-ethyl-Δ5-cholesten-3β-ol
Angelicin
Cinchol
Cupreol
Harzol
Quebrachol
Rhamnol
Sitosterin
Triastonal
α-dihydrofucosterol
α-phytosterol
Δ5-stigmasten-3β-ol

Star rating

5

What is it?

A plant sterol (phytosterol). There are over 40 known phytosterols but beta sitosterol is one of the most abundant being found in many plant oils, wheat germ and rice bran. Beta sitosterol is similar in structure to cholesterol (an animal sterol) since both are 4-desmethyl sterols (containing no methyl groups at carbon atom 4).

Claimed benefits

Reduces total and low-density lipoprotein (LDL) cholesterol levels and improves the symptoms of benign prostatic hyperplasia (BPH) such as improving urinary flow rate.

Deranged cholesterol values and exacerbation of BPH symptoms can be side effects of other anabolic/androgenic substances used by sports people.

Mode of Action

For cholesterol reduction beta sitosterol reduces absorption of cholesterol from the gut by up to 50% by competing with cholesterol to be incorporated into micelles. These are the microscopic transport packages via which fats are absorbed from the gut (1).

For relief from the symptoms of BPH the mechanism of action is unknown. It is known that beta sitosterol does not reduce prostate size so it must work via some other mechanism. One study has shown beta sitosterol has a significant effect on stromal TGFβ production within the prostate *in vitro* but more work is needed to confirm if this is responsible for its therapeutic effect (2).

Effectiveness

The ability of beta sitosterol to reduce serum total cholesterol and LDL cholesterol has been demonstrated in many human trials. A review of 14 randomized controlled trials (1) concluded that increasing reductions in LDL cholesterol levels are achieved with increasing amounts of beta sitosterol up to a maximum of 2g per day. Beyond 2g no additional benefit is seen. The review concluded that 2g/day of beta sitosterol reduces serum LDL concentrations by 14% for people aged 50-59, 9% for ages 40-49 and 11% for ages 30-39. In the 50-59 age group this reduces the risk of heart disease by 25% after about 2 years which the review comments "is as much as any cholesterol-lowering drug except statins."

These results have continued to be confirmed by trials carried out after the review (3) and beta sitosterol has also been shown to have similar benefits for younger people, reducing LDL levels 14.6% in a study involving young males with an average age of 24 (4).

The FDA authorized use of labelling health claims about the role of plant sterol or plant stanol esters in reducing the risk of coronary heart disease for foods containing these substances in the year 2000 (5).

The ability of beta sitosterol to improve symptomatic BPH has also been demonstrated by several human trials (6), (7). A systematic review of four of the largest and best designed trials using dosages from 60mg to 195mg/day reported an average improvement of 35% in symptoms compared to placebo (8).

A longer term study also found that improvements remained while continuing to take the beta sitosterol for up to 18 months (the duration of the study) (2).

Commonly used dosages

Beta sitosterol is often included in sport supplements in amounts from 100 to 250mg.

It is also sold as a stand alone supplement in a wide variety of formulations with quantities of 100mg up to 400mg being common.

For cholesterol reduction a dose of 2g per day is recommended.

For relief of BPH symptoms most of the studies above used doses from 20mg to 65mg three times a day.

Safety

No known safety issues.

Interactions

Ezetimibe, a drug which inhibits the intestinal absorption of cholesterol can also inhibit the absorption of beta sitosterol (9).

Statins, a class of drugs used to lower cholesterol levels may also lower serum levels of beta sitosterol. This has been seen with the drug pravastatin, but may also occur with other statins (10).

References

1. Law M. Plant sterol and stanol margarines and health. BMJ 2000;320:861-4.
2. Berges RR, Kassen A, Senge T. Treatment of symptomatic benign prostatic hyperplasia with beta-sitosterol: an 18-month follow-up. BJU Int 2000;85:842-6.
3. Neil HA, Meijer GW, Roe LS. Randomised controlled trial of use by hypercholesterolaemic patients of a vegetable oil sterol-enriched fat spread. Atherosclerosis 2001;156:329-37.
4. Matvienko OA, Lewis DS, Swanson M, Arndt B, Rainwater DL, Stewart J and Lee Alekel D. A single daily dose of soybean phytosterols in ground beef decreases serum total cholesterol and LDL cholesterol in young, mildly hypercholesterolemic men. Am J Clin Nutr 2002;76:57-64.
5. FDA Talkpaper: FDA Authorizes New Coronary Heart Disease Claim For Plant Sterol And Plant Stanol Esters [online] at

http://www.fda.gov/bbs/topics/ANSWERS/ANS01033.
html

6. Berges RR, Windeler J, Trampisch HJ, Senge T. Randomised, placebo-controlled, double-blind clinical trial of beta-sitosterol in patients with benign prostatic hyperplasia. Beta-sitosterol Study Group. Lancet 1995;345:1529-32.

7. Klippel KF, Hiltl DM, Schipp B. A multicentric, placebo-controlled, double-blind clinical trial of beta-sitosterol (phytosterol) for the treatment of benign prostatic hyperplasia. Br J Urol 1997;80:427-32.

8. Wilt TJ, MacDonald R, Ishani A. beta-sitosterol for the treatment of benign prostatic hyperplasia: a systematic review. BJU Int 1999;83:976-83.

9. Sudhop T, Lutjohann D, Kodal A, Igel M, Tribble DL, Shah S, *et al.* Inhibition of intestinal cholesterol absorption by ezetimibe in humans. Circulation 2002;106:1943-8.

10. Hidaka H, Kojima H, Kawabata T, Nakamura T, Konaka K, Kashiwagi A, *et al.* Effects of an HMG-CoA reductase inhibitor, pravastatin, and bile sequestering resin, cholestyramine, on plasma plant sterol levels in hypercholesterolemic subjects. J Atheroscler Thromb 1995;2:60-5.

Betaine

Other names

1-Carboxy-N,N,N-trimethylmethanaminium inner salt
(Carboxymethyl)trimethylammonium hydroxide inner salt
Abromine
Acidin-pepsin
Betaine anhydrous
Glycine betaine
Glycocoll betaine
Glycylbetaine
Jortaine
Lycine
Oxyneurine
Trimethylglycine
Trimethylglycocoll

Caution: Do not confuse with Betaine Hydrochloride.

Star rating

2

What is it?

Betaine is a methyl derivative of the amino acid glycine. Humans can either ingest betaine in the diet or it can be produced in the liver and kidneys via oxidation of choline. Betaine is found in many plant and animal foodstuffs and is present in high amounts in wheat, spinach, beets, pretzels and shrimp (1).

Claimed benefits

As a health supplement betaine is most often used to reduce circulating levels of the amino acid homocysteine since people with high plasma concentrations of homocysteine (called hyperhomocysteinemia or homocysteinemia) have increased risks of cardiovascular disease, stroke, Alzheimer's disease, dementia, and other metabolic disorders.

In sport supplements however betaine is usually added for three reasons;

Firstly as a "cell volumiser" by maintaining maximum hydration of cells. This has the cosmetic benefit of giving a pumped up appearance to musculature and it is also theorized that the stretching of the muscle fascia which this causes can induce or facilitate muscle hypertrophy.

Secondly in order to prevent dehydration and the consequent loss of performance that this causes during sporting activities.

Thirdly, betaine is frequently added to supplements containing glycocyamine. Glycocyamine is a creatine precursor which is converted to creatine in the liver and which is claimed to be effective even for creatine non-responders. However the process of converting glycocyamine to creatine in the liver depletes the liver of methyl groups which are necessary for the conversion of homocysteine to methionine. As we mentioned previously, high levels of homocysteine are related to cardiovascular disease and a range of other health problems. Betaine is added to prevent this hepatic depletion of methyl groups.

Mode of Action

As a hydration and cell volumising agent betaine synthesis is triggered in the mitochondria of cells when they are exposed to dehydration or temperature stress. Betaine is an osmolyte which increases cellular water retention, replaces inorganic salts, and protects intracellular enzymes against osmotic or temperature induced inactivation (1).

As a methyl donor in the conversion of glycocyamine betaine replaces methyl groups which are depleted by glycocyamine. Plasma levels of homocysteine are partly determined by the amount of homocysteine which is remethylated to methionine using the methyl-group of either 5-methyltetrahydrofolate or betaine which transfers a methyl group via the enzyme betaine homocysteine methyl transferase (2).

Effectiveness

There has been little research into the effectiveness of betaine as a cellular hydration agent. A small study on thoroughbred race horses indicated that betaine supplementation was effective at reducing plasma lactate concentrations during recovery from exercise in untrained horses but had no effect in trained horses (3). In small human studies involving male runners and performing resistance training, it was found that betaine produced no significant differences in hydration indices or performance and did not produce significant differences when added to carbohydrate sport drinks compared to a carbohydrate drink alone (4), (5), (6).

Betaine has been demonstrated effective at preventing glycocyamine induced rises in plasma homocysteine levels in studies on rats (2). However there are no studies indicating its effectiveness in humans or indicating an effective dose of betaine necessary to counteract a specific dose of glycocyamine.

When added to glycocyamine containing products betaine is frequently included in a betaine :glycocyamine ratio of 4:1 which is claimed to be the necessary ratio in order to make glycocyamine safe. This 4:1 ratio appears to originate in a patent filed by ME Boorsook who conducted research on glycocyamine in the 1950's. However I have been unable to discover any scientific rationale for this specific 4:1 ratio.

Commonly used dosages

Betaine is usually included as part of a proprietary formulation in commercial sport supplement preparations with the exact quantity of the substance not listed in the ingredients. When listed amounts from 500mg to 2000mg can be seen.

When sold as a stand alone product betaine is sold as a free powder or in capsules with a typical dose of 1000mg.

Safety

No known safety issues.

Interactions

None known.

References

1. Craig SAS, Betaine in Human Nutrition. Am J Clin Nutr 2004;80:539–49

2. Setoue M, Ohuchi S, Morita T, Sugiyama K. Hyperhomocysteinemia Induced by Guanidinoacetic Acid Is Effectively Suppressed by Choline and Betaine in Rats. Biosci. Biotechnol. Biochem 2008;72 (7):1696–1703

3. Warren LK, Lawrence LM, Thompson KN. The influence of betaine on untrained and trained horses exercising to fatigue. J Anim Sci 1999;77(3):677-684

4. Armstrong L E, Roti MW, Hatch HL, Sutherland JW, Mahood NV, Clements JM *et al.* Rehydration with fluids containing betaine: running performance and metabolism in a 31 degree C environment. Med Sci Sports Exerc 2005;35(5):Supplement S311

5. Maresh CM, Farrell MJ, Kraemer WJ, Yamamoto LM, Lee EC, Armstrong LE *et al.* The effects of betaine supplementation on strength and power performance. Med Sci Sports Exerc 2007;39(5):Supplement S101

6. Armstrong LE, Casa DJ, Roti MW, Lee EC, Craig SA, Sutherland JW *et al.* Influence of betaine consumption on strenuous running and sprinting in a hot environment. J Strength Cond Res. 2008;22(3):851-60.

Buchu

Other names

Agathosma betulina
Agathosma crenulata
Barosma betulina
Barosma crenulata
Barosma serratifolia
Bookoo
Bucco
Bucku
Diosma betulina
Parapetalifera betulina
Parapetalifera crenulata

Star rating

1

What is it?

A small South African shrub.

Claimed benefits

Diuretic.

Mode of Action

The principal active extract of the leaf is diosphenol (2-Hydroxy-3-methyl-6-(1-methylethyl)-2-cyclohexen-1-one) which is believed to act as a diuretic by causing irritation to the lining of the bladder and hence stimulating increased frequency of urination (1).

Effectiveness

No known data demonstrating effectiveness.

Commonly used dosages

As a liquid extract, 3.5g or 1/8th oz

As a solid extract, 1g or 1/30 oz (2).

Safety

Contains pulegone, a potential hepatotoxin (3) and so should be avoided in liver disease.

May cause renal irritation and so should be avoided in kidney disease (4).

May increase menstrual bleeding or provoke miscarriage (1).

Interactions

It is believed that Buchu may have anticoagulant properties. If taken together with anticoagulant/antiplatelet drugs, the time taken to stop bleeding may be increased (5).

References

1. Drug Digest [online] at http://www.drugdigest.org/DD/DVH/HerbsWho/0,392 3,4085%7CBuchu,00.html
2. Grieve, M. *Botanical.com* [online] at http://www.botanical.com/botanical/mgmh/b/buchu-78.html

3. De Smet PAGM, Keller K, Hansel R, Chandler RF. eds. Adverse Effects of Herbal Drugs, vol 2. Berlin: Springer-Verlag; 1993
4. Barnes J, Anderson LA, Phillipson JD. Herbal Medicines 3rd Edition. London & Chicago: Pharmaceutical Press; 2007
5. Fetrow CW, Avila JR. Professional's Handbook of Complementary & Alternative Medicines. 1st ed. Springhouse, PA: Springhouse Corp; 1999

Caffeine

Other names

1,3,7-trimethyl-2,6-dioxopurine
1,3,7-trimethylpurine-2,6-dione
1,3,7-Trimethylxanthine
3,7-Dihydro-1,3,7-trimethyl-1H-purine-2,6-dione
Cafeina
Coffeine
Guaranine
Koffein
Mateina
Methyltheobromine
Thein
Theine

Star rating

5

What is it?

A naturally occuring purine alkaloid present in coffee beans, tea and some other plants.

Claimed benefits

A stimulant, increases endurance and exercise intensity. Fat loss.

Mode of Action

Caffeine has a stimulant effect on the central nervous system. It achieves this by preventing the inhibitory substance adenosine from binding to $\alpha 1$ and $\alpha 2A$ receptors on nerves. Adenosine is a substance produced in the body to help control the responsiveness of nerves to neurotransmitters (1).

The analgesic effects of caffeine via increased secretion of β-endorphins may reduce perception of pain and blunt perceived exertion during exercise which could partially prevent inhibition of motor units leading to greater muscle contraction and force production (2).

Effectiveness

The effectiveness of caffeine in improving aerobic type endurance sport performance has been clearly demonstrated and accepted by scientists. Improvements of approximately 3% in performance are obtained when 3 – 9mg/kg of caffeine are taken before or during exercise (3) (4) (5). No additional benefit is obtained from doses above 9mg/kg and caffeine exerts a greater ergogenic effect on performance if consumed in an anhydrous state (i.e. as a pure caffeine supplement) rather than coffee. This may be because other compounds present in coffee such as chlorogenic acids reduce the ability of caffeine to inhibit adenosine (6).

For anaerobic exercise type sport or resistance training while the evidence is not as clear cut as for aerobic activity, on balance the evidence is in favour of the fact that caffeine supplementation can also improve performance. In a recent systematic review (7) of all available studies, 11 out of 17 studies showed significant performance improvements in power based sports and 6 out of 11 studies showed significant benefits of caffeine for resistance training.

Caffeine appears to have maximal effect in those people who do not regularly consume caffeine or in those who have abstained from it for at least 7 days (3).

Finally, for weight loss although caffeine increases lipolysis and thermogenesis (6) multiple studies have failed to convincingly show that caffeine is effective for weight loss when taken alone. Nevertheless it does act synergistically with other weight loss agents such as ephedra (8) and nicotine (9) increasing their weight loss effect. How this works is not completely understood.

Commonly used dosages

Caffeine is often included as part of a proprietary formulation in commercial sport supplement preparations with the exact quantity of the substance not listed in the ingredients. However when listed amounts between 100mg and 200mg are most common.

In the studies which showed a proven weight loss effect from caffeine and ephedra an ephedrine/caffeine combination of 20mg/200mg three times a day was usually used (note: ephedra supplements are not legally available in all countries due to safety concerns).

A standard cup of coffee provides around 100mg of caffeine.

Safety

Caffeine is safe when consumed in normal amounts found in food and drinks or when taken as a supplement at the recommended doses, although minor effects such as nervousness or insomnia may be experienced.

However when taken in overdose caffeine can have serious adverse effects including death. These include nausea, vomiting, tremors, high blood pressure, irregular and rapid heart beat and convulsions among others (1).

Never exceed the stated dose.

Concerns that caffeine may cause dehydration affecting either health or peformance during exercise do not appear to be supported by the current evidence (6).

Interactions

Caffeine may increase the side effects from beta adrenergic drugs such as the asthma medicines albuterol or salbutamol. It can also increase the risk of toxicity from the drug clozapine (used in the treatment of schizophrenia) by increasing blood levels of the drug. Conversely it can reduce blood levels of the drug lithium reducing its effectiveness.

Caffeine can also enhance the effects of acetaminophen (paracetamol) and aspirin (1).

There is a theoretical possibility that caffeine may interact with a wide variety of other medications, effects are likely to be small at normal intakes of caffeine but if you are concerned you should consult your doctor.

References

1. Oregon State University. Linus Pauling Institute. Micronutrient Informtion Center. Coffee. [online] at http://lpi.oregonstate.edu/infocenter/foods/coffee/
2. Davis JK, Green JM. Caffeine and anaerobic performance: ergogenic value and mechanisms of action. Sports Med. 2009;39(10):813-32
3. Ganio MS, Klau JF, Casa DJ, Armstrong LE, Maresh CM. Effect of caffeine on sport-specific endurance performance: a systematic review. J Strength Cond Res. 2009;23(1):315-24
4. Kreider RB, Wilborn CD, Taylor L, Campbell B, Almada AL *et al.* ISSN exercise & sport nutrition review: research & recommendations. J Int Soc Sports Nutr. 2010;7:7
5. Cox GR, Desbrow B, Montgomery PG, Anderson ME, Bruce CR *et al.* Effect of different protocols of caffeine intake on metabolism and endurance performance. J Appl Physiol. 2002;93(3):990-9
6. Goldstein ER, Ziegenfuss T, Kalman D, Kreider R, Campbell B *et al.* International society of sports nutrition position stand: caffeine and performance. J Int Soc Sports Nutr. 2010;7(1):5
7. Astorino TA, Roberson DW. Efficacy of acute caffeine ingestion for short-term high-intensity exercise performance: a systematic review. J Strength Cond Res. 2010;24(1):257-65
8. Diepvens K, Westerterp KR, Westerterp-Plantenga MS. Obesity and thermogenesis related to the consumption of caffeine, ephedrine, capsaicin, and green tea. Am J Physiol Regul Integr Comp Physiol. 2007;292(1):R77-85. Epub 2006 Jul 13
9. Jessen A, Buemann B, Toubro S, Skovgaard IM, Astrup A. The appetite-suppressant effect of nicotine is enhanced by caffeine. Diabetes Obes Metab. 2005;7(4):327-33

Calcium D-Glucarate

Other names

Calcium Glucarate
Calcium-D Glucarate
Calcium-D-Glucarate
D-glucaro-1,4-lactone (1,4 GL)

Star rating

2

What is it?

Calcium-D-glucarate is the calcium salt of D-glucaric acid which is a natural substance found in various foodstuffs with the highest concentrations being found in oranges, apples, brussel sprouts, broccoli, and cabbage (1).

Claimed benefits

Aids in the elimination of estrogen from the body and reduces serum estrogen levels.
Increases serum testosterone levels (via reduced negative feedback from estrogen to the pituitary gland).

Mode of Action

In the acidic environment of the stomach approximately one third of calcium d-glucarate is converted into glucaro-1,4-lactone which is an inhibitor of the enzyme β-glucuronidase.

As part of the elimination of the hormone estrogen from the human body it is conjugated with glucuronic acid in the liver to an insoluble form which is excreted into the intestines and eliminated from the body. However some of the naturally occurring bacteria in the bowel produce the enzyme β-glucuronidase which breaks down the bond between estrogen and glucuronic acid converting estrogen back into a soluble form which can be reabsorbed from the bowel back into the circulation.

By inhibiting the enzyme β-glucuronidase, calcium d-glucarate reduces the amount of estrogen which can be reabsorbed (2).

Effectiveness

The ability of orally consumed calcium d-glucarate to inhibit β-glucuronidase activity both in the blood and in various body tissues such as liver, lung and intestines has been demonstrated by *in vivo* experiments on rats (1). There is also evidence from rat studies that this does lead to a reduction in endogenous levels of estrogen (3).

However, no studies have been performed to determine the extent of this effect in humans or what effective dose of calcium d-glucarate would be necessary to achieve it.

Commonly used dosages

Calcium D-glucarate is often included in sports supplements in amounts of 200-300mg together with various other compounds. It is also sold as a stand alone supplement in capsules or tablets ranging from 200mg to 500mg.

Safety

No known safety issues. Calcium D-glutarate was not seen to exert any adverse effects on rats even when it composed 10% of their total diet by weight (1).

Interactions

None known.

References

1. Dwivedi C, Heck WJ, Downie AA, Larroya S, Webb TE. Effect of calcium glucarate on B-glucuronidase activity and glucarate content on certain vegetables and fruits. Biochem Med Metab Bio 1990;43:83-92.
2. Douglas C. Hall, M.D. Nutritional Influence on Estrogen Metabolism by Applied Nutritional Science Reports, 2001 (article) available online at http://www.cabecahealth.com/PDF%20files/NutrInfluencesEstrogen.pdf
3. Walaszek Z, Hanausek-Walaszek M, Minton JP, Webb TE. Dietary glucarate as anti-promter of 7,12-dimethylbenz(a)anthracene-induced mammary tumorigenesis. Carcinogenesis 1986;7:1463-6.

Capsaicin

Other names

Capsicum
Capsicutin
Cayenne pepper
Chilli pepper
Civamide
Isodecanoic acid vanillylamide
Oleoresin Capsicum
Paprika
Red pepper

Trans-8-methyl-N-vanillyl-6-nonenamide, N-(4-Hydroxy-3-methoxyphenyl)-8-methyl-non-trans-6-enamide (E)-N-[(4-hydroxy-3-methoxyphenyl)methyl]-8-methylnon-6-enamide

Star rating

4

What is it?

Capsaicin is a phytochemical (an alkylamide) having the molecular formula $C_{18}H_{27}NO_3$ which is found in the genus of plants capsicum. Capsicum is native to South America, India and other tropical countries and is cultivated worldwide. It contains approximately 0.11% capsaicinoids (depending on the species) of which capsaicin is the major component, but it also contains the other capsaicinoids dihydrocapsaicin, nordihydrocapsaicin, homodihydrocapsaicin and homocapsaicin (1).

Claimed benefits

Weight loss.

Mode of Action

Capsaicin induces thermogenesis (increased heat production) in humans via stimulation of the symapathetic nervous system and enhanced catecholamine (stimulatory hormones such as adrenaline and noradrenaline) secretion from the adrenal medulla (2), (3), (4), (5) which stimulates gluconeogenesis and lipolysis. This thermogenesis is probably mediated by β-adrenergic stimulation since it is prevented by the administration of a β-adrenergic blocker such as propranolol (2).

Capsaicin also increases the rate of body heat loss hence increasing the total amount of calories used by the body (5) and reduces total food intake by causing both a reduction in appetite (6), (7), (8) and a switch in eating behaviour to eat less carbohydrate and fat but not affecting total protein intake (6), (7). This is caused by the ability of capsaicin to activate appetite regulating neurons and neuropeptides (9).

These effects of capsaicin appear to be largely unrelated to its spicy flavour or local heat sensation in the mouth since the ingestion of pepper or capsaicin capsules has a similar effect (7), (10).

Effectiveness

The studies outlined above have shown the ability of capsaicin to suppress appetite and reduce total energy intake from food between approximately 8% to 11%.

Capsaicin has been shown to induce thermogenesis and increase body temperature by 0.2-0.3 degrees centigrade (5).

However no studies have been performed to discover how this equates to weight loss or body composition changes and more research is needed to quantify these effects.

Although normally considered as a thermogenic agent, the ability of capsaicin to increase catecholamine secretion and stimulate the sympathetic nervous system also classifies it as a stimulant. Although again further studies are needed to quantify this effect.

Commonly used dosages

Capsaicin is usually included in commercial sport supplements in the form of cayenne or red pepper which is usually included as part of a proprietary formulation with the exact quantity of the substance not listed in the ingredients.

When the quantity of cayenne pepper is listed there is a wide variation in amounts included from 50mg to 500mg.

In the studies quoted above a wide variety of quantities of pepper were used from 3g/day up to 12g/day containing between 2.5mg/g and 3mg/g of capsaicin.

Safety

Capsicum is known to induce various gastrointestinal cancers in test animals such as rats and mice when fed to them at high concentrations but there are no known links to cancer in humans at normal levels of intake. Capsicum is generally recognized as safe by the U.S. Food and Drug Administration for use in food (11).

Interactions

There is a small theoretical risk that capsaicin could potentiate the effect of anti-platelet drugs such as aspirin, clopidogrel and dipyridamole increasing the risk of bruising and bleeding (12), (13).

References

1. Barnes J, Anderson LA, Phillipson JD. Herbal Medicines 3rd Ed. London, Pharmaceutical Press, 2007.
2. Yoshioka M, Lim K, Kikuzato S, Kiyonnaga A, Tanaka H, Shindo M, Suzuki M. Effects of red-pepper diet on the energy metabolism in men. J Nutr Sci Vitaminol (Tokyo). 1995;41(6):647-56
3. Yoshioka M, St-Pierre S, Suzuki M, Tremblay A. Effects of red pepper added to high-fat and high-carbohydrate

meals on energy metabolism and substrate utilization in Japanese women. Br J Nutr 1998;80:503-510

4. Lim K, Yoshioka M, Kikuzato S, Kiyonaga A, Tanaka H, Shindo M *et al.* Dietary red pepper ingestion increases carbohydrate oxidation at rest and during exercise in runners. Med Sci Sports Exerc. 1997;29(3):355-61

5. Hachiya S, Kawabata F, Ohnuki K, Inoue N, Yoneda H, Yazawa S *et al.* Effects of CH-19 Sweet, a non-pungent cultivar of red pepper, on sympathetic nervous activity, body temperature, heart rate, and blood pressure in humans. Biosci Biotechnol Biochem. 2007;71(3):671-6.

6. Yoshioka M, St-Pierre S, Drapeau V, Dionne I, Doucet E, Suzuki M *et al.* Effects of red pepper on appetite and energy intake. Br J Nutr. 1999;82(2):115-23

7. Westerterp-Plantenga MS, Smeets A, Lejeune MP. Sensory and gastrointestinal satiety effects of capsaicin on food intake. Int J Obes (Lond). 2005;29(6):682-8

8. Yoshioka M, Doucet E, Drapeau V, Dionne I, Tremblay A. Combined effects of red pepper and caffeine consumption on 24 h energy balance in subjects given free access to foods. Br J Nutr. 2001;85(2):203-11

9. Buck SH, Burks TF. The neuropharmacology of capsaicin: review of some recent observations. Pharmacol Rev. 1986;38(3):179-226

10. Yoshioka M, Imanaga M, Ueyama H, Yamane M, Kubo Y, Boivin A *et al.* Maximum tolerable dose of red pepper decreases fat intake independently of spicy sensation in the mouth. Br J Nutr. 2004;91(6):991-5

11. Final report on the safety assessment of capsicum annuum extract, capsicum annuum fruit extract, capsicum annuum resin, capsicum annuum fruit powder, capsicum frutescens fruit, capsicum frutescens fruit extract, capsicum frutescens resin, and capsaicin. Int J Toxicol. 2007;26 Suppl 1:3-106

12. Hogaboam CM, Wallace JL. Inhibition of platelet aggregation by capsaicin. An effect unrelated to actions

on sensory afferent neurons. Eur J Pharmacol 1991;202:129-31.
13. Wang JP, Hsu MF, Teng CM. Antiplatelet effect of capsaicin. Thromb Res 1984;36:497-507.

Cassia Cinnamon

Other names

Batavia Cassia
Canton cassia
Cassia
Cassia aromaticum
Cassia bark
Chinese cinnamon
Cinnamomum aromaticum
Cinnamomum cassia
Padang-Cassia

Caution: Do not confuse with other forms of cinnamon. Cinnamomum verum (Ceylon cinnamon) is also often sold however Cassia cinnamon was used in the original studies investigating the effect of cinnamon on insulin sensitivity and so is the type commonly included in sport supplements. Cinnamomum verum also contains the compound thought to cause the increase in insulin sensitivity but in lesser quantities (1).

A commercial product called Cinulin PF ® is available and is used in many sport supplements. This is an extract produced from Cinnamomum burmannii a related species which is claimed to be standardized for the doubly linked Type-A Polymers which are the compounds which affect insulin sensitivity.

Star rating

4

What is it?

A small evergreen tree of the Lauraceae family native to Sri Lanka. The bark is commonly used as a spice to flavour foods.

Claimed benefits

Weight loss.

Mode of Action

Water-soluble polyphenol polymers have been isolated from cinnamon. Nuclear magnetic resonance and mass spectroscopy analysis indicates their structure to be A type doubly linked procyanidin oligomers of the catechins and/or epicatechins. These polymers were found to have insulin enhancing effects by acting at the insulin receptor which may help to lower blood glucose and insulin levels (2).

Effectiveness

We can consider the effectiveness of cinnamon by looking at studies carried out both on type II diabetics and on healthy individuals.

In Type II diabetics there is conflicting evidence of the effectiveness of cinnamon at controlling blood sugar levels.

Three relatively large studies (3), (4), (5) showed that cinnamon was modestly effective at reducing blood glucose levels in type II diabetics. For example in a study (3) involving 60 people (equal numbers of men and women) subjects took either 1g, 3g or 6g of cinnamon daily spread over the day or a placebo. Blood glucose was analyzed at 0, 20, 40 and 60 days. After 20 days blood glucose was lower only in the group taking 6g. After 40 days fasting blood glucose was reduced between 18% to 29% with no significant difference between the groups taking 1g, 3g or 6g. Another double blind study involving 79 subjects found that taking 3g of cinnamon for four months reduced fasting blood glucose by 10.3% (5).

However in a further study involving 43 people and taking 1g of cinnamon for 3 months no effect on blood glucose was found (6).

Two systematic reviews of these studies have been conducted which attempt to statistically analyze all the data by combining the studies to obtain a greater sample size and hence gain greater accuracy. One of these systematic reviews (7) concluded that there was strong evidence for an effect of cinnamon on blood glucose while a second concluded that there were no statistically significant changes in blood glucose as a result of cinnamon (8). However the authors of this review admitted that their sample size may have been too small for the statistical method that they used.

On balance it seems likely that cinnamon does have some effect on blood glucose especially when we also consider the various studies carried out using healthy adults which were not included in the meta analyses above. These have shown that cinnamon used at doses of 3g and above (3g was the most common dose tested in these experiments) is capable of lowering blood glucose and the insulin response after meals by a statistically significant amount (9), (10), (11), (12).

Finally in a study (13) using 500mg/day of the commercial

cinnamon extract Cinnulin PF ® on 22 individuals with the metabolic syndrome (pre-diabetes) for a period of 12 weeks it was found that in addition to statistically significant falls in fasting blood glucose of 8.4% the subjects also experienced small, but statistically significant decreases in body fat of 0.7% and increases in lean mass of 1.1%.

Commonly used dosages

Cinnamon is often included as part of a proprietary formulation in commercial sport supplement preparations with the exact quantity of the substance not listed in the ingredients.

When the amount is listed quantities of 20mg, 75mg and 150mg have been seen in different products.

When sold as a stand alone supplement capsules from 125mg to 600mg are available.

As noted above, most of the studies showing an effect on blood glucose used amounts of 3g/daily. Greater effects were not seen with amounts above 3g.

Safety

In the USA cinnamon is listed as GRA (generally recognised as safe) by the FDA. The Council of Europe recognizes it as a natural food flavouring (14).

The German Federal Institute for Risk Assessment has issued a warning that Cassia cinnamon only (not other types of cinnamon such as Cinnamomum verum or Cinnamomum burmannii) may contain high levels of the compound coumarin which can cause elevation of liver enzymes and in severe cases inflammation of the liver. These effects are reversible on stopping coumarin ingestion (15).

There is one report of oral cinnamon supplementation causing a severe exacerbation of pre-existing rosacea in an individual suffering from this skin condition (16).

Interactions

Due to its effect on blood sugar and insulin, cinnamon may affect the performance of diabetes drugs leading to a risk of hypoglycemia.

References

1. Verspohl EJ, Bauer K, Neddermann E. Antidiabetic effect of Cinnamomum cassia and Cinnamomum zeylanicum in vivo and in vitro. Phytother Res 2005;19:203-6.
2. Anderson RA, Broadhurst CL, Polansky MM, Schmidt WF, Khan A, Flanagan VP *et al*. Isolation and characterization of polyphenol type-A polymers from cinnamon with insulin-like biological activity. J Agric Food Chem. 2004;52(1):65-70
3. Khan A, Safdar M, Ali Khan MM, Khattak KN, Anderson RA. Cinnamon improves glucose and lipids of people with type 2 diabetes. Diabetes Care. 2003;26(12):3215-8
4. Safdar M, Khan A, Khattak MMAK, Mohammad Siddique M. Effect of Various Doses of Cinnamon on Blood Glucose in Diabetic Individuals. Pakistan Journal of Nutrition 2004:3 (5): 268-272
5. Mang B, Wolters M, Schmitt B, Kelb K, Lichtinghagen R. *et al*. Effects of a cinnamon extract on plasma glucose, HbA, and serum lipids in diabetes mellitus type 2. Eur J Clin Invest. 2006;36(5):340-4
6. Blevins SM, Leyva MJ, Brown J, Wright J, Scofield RH, Aston CE. Effect of cinnamon on glucose and lipid levels

in non insulin-dependent type 2 diabetes. Diabetes Care. 2007;30(9):2236-7. Epub 2007 Jun 11

7. Dugoua JJ, Seely D, Perri D, Cooley K, Forelli T. *et al.* From type 2 diabetes to antioxidant activity: a systematic review of the safety and efficacy of common and cassia cinnamon bark. Can J Physiol Pharmacol. 2007;85(9):837-47

8. Baker WL, Gutierrez-Williams G, White CM, Kluger J, Coleman CI. Effect of cinnamon on glucose control and lipid parameters. Diabetes Care. 2008;31(1):41-3. Epub 2007 Oct 1

9. Solomon TP, Blannin AK. Changes in glucose tolerance and insulin sensitivity following 2 weeks of daily cinnamon ingestion in healthy humans. Eur J Appl Physiol. 2009;105(6):969-76. Epub 2009 Jan 22

10. Hlebowicz J, Hlebowicz A, Lindstedt S, Björgell O, Höglund P. *et al.* Effects of 1 and 3 g cinnamon on gastric emptying, satiety, and postprandial blood glucose, insulin, glucose-dependent insulinotropic polypeptide, glucagon-like peptide 1, and ghrelin concentrations in healthy subjects. Am J Clin Nutr. 2009;89(3):815-21. Epub 2009 Jan 21

11. Solomon TP, Blannin AK. Effects of short-term cinnamon ingestion on in vivo glucose tolerance. Diabetes Obes Metab. 2007;9(6):895-901

12. Hlebowicz J, Darwiche G, Björgell O, Almér LO. Effect of cinnamon on postprandial blood glucose, gastric emptying, and satiety in healthy subjects. Am J Clin Nutr. 2007;85(6):1552-6

13. Ziegenfuss TN, Hofheins JE, Mendel RW, Landis J, Anderson RA. Effects of a water-soluble cinnamon extract on body composition and features of the metabolic syndrome in pre-diabetic men and women. J Int Soc Sports Nutr. 2006;3:45-53

14. Barnes J, Anderson LA, Phillipson JD. Herbal Medicines. 3rd ed. London: Pharmaceutical Press; 2007

15. Selected Questions about coumarin in cinnamon and other foods. Federal Institute for Risk Assessment. [online] at http://www.bfr.bund.de/cd/8487
16. Campbell TM, Neems R, Moore J. Severe exacerbation of rosacea induced by cinnamon supplements. J Drugs Dermatol. 2008;7(6):586-7

Cayaponia Tayuya

Other names

Abobrinha do Mato
Anapinta
Bryonia tayuya
Cayaponia piauhiensis
Trianosperma ficifolia

Star rating

2

What is it?

A woody vine belonging to the Cucurbitaceae (gourd) family and native to the South American rainforest, particularly Brazil, Peru and Bolivia. It is used in the traditional medicine of native South American Indians and was recorded in the *Brazilian Pharmacopoeia* as an official herbal drug in 1929. It has many claimed benefits including analgesic, anti-inflammatory, anti-epileptic, anti-diarrheal, anti-cancer, treatment for irritable bowel syndrome, dyspepsia, eczema etc. (1)

Claimed benefits

Appetite stimulant and digestive aid.
Adaptogen.

Mode of Action

Various phytochemicals can be extracted from Cayaponia Tayuya including various flavones, glucosides and cucurbitacin triterpenes. One of these, cucurbitacin R diglucoside is believed to exert adaptogenic effects by stimulating the adrenal glands to moderately increase corticosteroid secretion in response to stress (2).

There is no known data regarding a mode of action as an appetite stimulant.

Effectiveness

The ability of Cayaponia Tayuya to exert adaptogenic effects on metabolism has been observed in several studies both *in vitro* and *in vivo* on rats (2), (3).

There is no known evidence regarding its effectiveness as an appetite stimulant.

Commonly used dosages

Cayaponia Tayuya is usually included as part of a proprietary formulation in commercial sport supplement preparations with the exact quantity of the substance not listed in the ingredients.

When sold as a stand alone supplement it is usually supplied in the form of a tea or as a liquid extract of the plant in alcohol.

In traditional medicine 1-2g of root powder are taken 2-3 times a day (4).

Safety

No known safety issues. Reported not to be toxic orally at doses up to 2000mg/kg (4).

Interactions

None known.

References

1. Raintree Nutrition. Tropical Plant Database [online] at http://www.rain-tree.com/tayuya.htm
2. Panossian A, Gabrielian E, Wagner H. On the mechanism of action of plant adaptogens with particular reference to cucurbitacin R diglucoside. Phytomedicine. 1999;6(3):147-55
3. Panosian AG, Dadaian MA, Gevorkian GA. Action of adaptogens: cucurbitacin R diglucoside as a stimulator of arachidonic acid metabolism in the rat adrenal gland. Probl Endokrinol (Mosk). 1989;35(2):70-4
4. James A Duke. Duke's Handbook of Medicinal Plants of Latin America. 1st Ed. Boca Raton: CRC Press; 2008.

Chasteberry

Other names

Agnus castus
Chaste tree
Mang Jing Zi
Monk's pepper
Sage tree hemp
Vitex
Vitex agnus-castus

Star rating

3

What is it?

A flowering shrub of the Lamiaceae family (formerly classified as part of Verbenaceae family) which grows in warm temperate and subtropical regions. It has been used throughout history as a traditional medicine in various cultures for the treatment of a variety of ailments, mainly those involving disorders of the female reproductive system. It was also used by medieval monks to reduce sexual desire and aid in the maintenance of their vows of chastity (1).

The German Commission E has approved its internal use for the treatment of menstrual complaints and irregularity as well as for mastodynia (breast pain) (2).

Claimed benefits

It is believed that some anabolic steroids cause gynecomastia (growth of breast tissue in males) by causing rises in the levels of the hormone prolactin which induces lobuloalveolar growth of the mammary gland. Chasteberry is claimed to be able to prevent or help control such side effects by reducing levels of prolactin.

Some also claim that chasteberry can raise testosterone levels.

Mode of Action

The hormone prolactin is secreted by the anterior pituitary gland. The amount secreted is controlled by a part of the brain called the hypothalamus. The hypothalamus produces a neurotransmitter called dopamine which suppresses the release of prolactin from the pituitary gland. Various other hormones are involved in the control of prolactin such as estrogen, thyroid releasing hormone and gonadotropin releasing hormone (3), but only dopamine is relevant to our discussion of chasteberry.

Certain compounds found in chasteberry are able to bind to dopamine receptors and hence have the action of dopamine in the pituitary gland to suppress prolactin secretion. These compounds are known as diterpines of which five exert over 50% of the dopaminergic activity of chasteberry. These five have the structure cleroda-x,14-dien-13-ol (molecular weight 290) and so are called clerodadienols. The clerodadienols appear to have a potency approximately equivalent to that of dopamine in preventing prolactin release when present at concentrations 50 times higher than dopamine (4).

Effectiveness

Most of the research involving chasteberry has involved evaluation of menstrual symptoms and few studies have looked directly at its effect on prolactin levels.

In women two studies (5), (6) were found which demonstrated that chasteberry was effective at lowering prolactin levels in women suffering from latent hyperprolactinaemia (high prolactin levels not due to a pituitary adenoma). In one of these studies (6) involving 40 women, 40mg daily of chasteberry was found to be as effective at lowering prolactin as the dopamine agonist drug bromocriptine.

In the only known study involving men the effect of chasteberry appeared to be dose dependent. At doses of 120mg/day prolactin levels were increased in the 20 men in the study, however at doses of 240mg/day and 480mg/day there was a modest reduction in prolactin levels.

There was no significant effect on testosterone levels in this study.

Commonly used dosages

Chasteberry is supplied in a wide variety of strengths from 40mg to 500mg.

Safety

A systematic review of the safety of chasteberry concluded that there are no serious safety issues. Mild adverse reactions include nausea, headache, gastrointestinal disturbances and rashes (7).

Interactions

Due to its ability to bind to the dopamine receptor chasteberry may theoretically interact with both dopamine agonist and antagonist drugs either potentiating or reducing their effect.

Examples of dopamine agonist drugs are bromocriptine and levodopa. Examples of dopamine antagonist drugs are antipsychotic drugs such as chlorpromazine, clozapine, fluphenazine and haloperidol. It would be wise to avoid taking chasteberry if on any of these classes of medication.

References

1. Tracy TS, Kingston RL. Herbal Products Toxicology and Clinical Pharmacology. 2nd ed. New Jersey: Humana Press; 2007
2. Barnes J, Anderson LA, Phillipson JD. Herbal Medicines. 3rd ed. London: Pharmaceutical Press; 2007
3. Bowen R, Prolactin [online] Available at http://arbl.cvmbs.colostate.edu/hbooks/pathphys/endo crine/hypopit/prolactin.html
4. Wuttke W, Jarry H, Christoffel V, Spengler B, Seidlová-Wuttke D. Chaste tree (Vitex agnus-castus)--pharmacology and clinical indications. Phytomedicine. 2003;10(4):348-57.
5. Milewicz A, Gejdel E, Sworen H, Sienkiewicz K, Jedrzejak J, Teucher T, Schmitz H. Vitex agnus castus extract in the treatment of luteal phase defects due to latent hyperprolactinemia. Results of a randomized placebo-controlled double-blind study. Arzneimittelforschung. 1993;43(7):752-6
6. Kilicdag EB, Tarim E, Bagis T, Erkanli S, Aslan E, Ozsahin K, Kuscu E. Fructus agni casti and bromocriptine for treatment of hyperprolactinemia and mastalgia. Int J Gynaecol Obstet. 2004;85(3):292-3
7. Daniele C, Thompson Coon J, Pittler MH, Ernst E. Vitex agnus castus: a systematic review of adverse events. Drug Saf. 2005;28(4):319-32

Choline

Other names

(β-hydroxyethyl)trimethylammonium
2-hydroxyethyl(trimethyl)azanium
2-Hydroxy-N,N,N-trimethylethanaminium
Bilineurine
Choline Bitartrate
Choline Chloride
Choline Citrate
Cholinum
L-Choline
Methylated phosphatidylethanolamine
Trimethylethanolamine

Star rating

1

What is it?

Choline is an organic compound having the molecular formula $C_5H_{14}NO^+$ and traditionally considered as one of the B vitamins. It is no longer regarded as such since we now know that choline can be synthesized by the human body in the liver via the methylation of phosphatidylethanolamine.

It is nevertheless classified as an essential nutrient since the quantity produced in the body is insufficient to maintain health and choline must be consumed in the diet. Choline deficiency is rare but can result in liver damage.

Choline rich foods are liver, beef, wheat germ, egg, cod, broccoli and brussel sprouts. No RDA (recommended dietary allowance) has been set for choline however the US Food and

Nutrition Board has set an Adequate Intake level for the prevention of liver damage as 550mg/day for men and 425mg/day for women (1).

Claimed benefits

Delays fatigue in endurance sports.

Aids fat loss when combined with carnitine.

Mode of Action

It was observed that those undertaking endurance sports suffered falls in the level of plasma choline. For example one study found that marathon runners experienced a 40% reduction in the level of plasma choline after a marathon (2). Such reductions are associated with reduced acetylcholine release from the neuromuscular junction since choline is a precursor for acetylcholine (acetylcholine is a neurotransmitter necessary for muscle function). It was postulated that choline supplementation would prevent this and delay the onset of fatigue.

For fat loss, choline has been shown to conserve carnitine by increasing its uptake by the tissues possibly by upregulating the sodium-dependent carnitine transporter (OCTN 2) which is present in most tissues. This produces enhanced fatty acid oxidation (3).

Effectiveness

Various studies have investigated the effect of choline supplementation during intense and endurance exercise conditions but found no benefit to performance or perceived exhaustion (4), (5), (6).

In a study involving 19 women receiving 0.94g/day of choline and 0.68g/day of carnitine or placebo over three weeks with both groups undertaking light aerobic exercise 3-5 days a week, biochemical markers indicated that carnitine was preserved and that enhanced fatty acid oxidation was occurring. However while both the placebo and choline plus carnitine groups lost weight over the study period there was no statistical difference between them. Furthermore, while both groups lost weight there was no reduction in body fat percentage indicating that neither group had preferentially lost fat rather than lean muscle tissue (3).

In a study using rats a combination of caffeine, carnitine and choline was found to reduce body fat more than rats receiving no supplements however the difference was not statistically significant. This study also gave the rats an amount of choline equivalent to 800mg/kg of body weight. For a 70 kg human this would be equivalent to consuming 56g an amount far in excess of the recommended upper safe limit of 3.5g. Also the researchers did not test the caffeine separately so it is not possible to discount any individual effect of the caffeine (7).

Commonly used dosages

Choline is included in sports supplements in a wide variety of quantities with amounts from 75mg to 300mg being common. It is usually included in weight loss supplements with a variety of other ingredients.

As a stand alone supplement it is commonly sold as tablets or capsules ranging in strength from 250mg to 500mg.

Safety

The upper safe daily limit has been set at 3.5g by the US

Food and Nutrition Board. Amounts over this can cause a fishy body odour, nausea, vomiting and low blood pressure which may result in dizzines or fainting (1).

Interactions

Individuals taking the drug methotrexate may have an increased requirement for choline (1).

References

1. Choline. Linus Pauling Institute [online] at http://lpi.oregonstate.edu/infocenter/othernuts/choline/
2. Conlay LA, Sabounjian LA, Wurtman RJ. Exercise and neuromodulators: choline and acetylcholine in marathon runners. Int J Sports Med. 1992;13 Suppl 1:S141-2
3. Hongu N, Sachan DS. Carnitine and choline supplementation with exercise alter carnitine profiles, biochemical markers of fat metabolism and serum leptin concentration in healthy women. J Nutr. 2003;133(1):84-9
4. Warber JP, Patton JF, Tharion WJ, Zeisel SH, Mello RP *et al.* The effects of choline supplementation on physical performance. Int J Sport Nutr Exerc Metab. 2000;10(2):170-81
5. Spector SA, Jackman MR, Sabounjian LA, Sakkas C, Landers DM, Willis WT. Effect of choline supplementation on fatigue in trained cyclists. Med Sci Sports Exerc. 1995;27(5):668-73
6. Deuster PA, Singh A, Coll R, Hyde DE, Becker WJ. Choline ingestion does not modify physical or cognitive performance. Mil Med. 2002;167(12):1020-5
7. Hongu N, Sachan DS. Caffeine, carnitine and choline supplementation of rats decreases body fat and serum

leptin concentration as does exercise. J Nutr. 2000;130(2):152-7

Chromium

Other names

Chromic Chloride
Chromium Acetate
Chromium Chloride
Chromium III
Chromium Nicotinate
Chromium Picolinate
Chromium Polynicotinate
Chromium Trichloride
Chromium Tripicolinate
Trivalent Chromium

Star rating

1

What is it?

An essential trace mineral which exists in a number of forms. The most common form found in food and used by the human body is chromium III. Chromium is found in many foods particularly brocolli, grape juice, potatoes, apples and bananas. The US Food and Nutrition Board has set an adequate intake of chromium at 35 mcg/day for men and 30 mcg/day for women (1).

Sport supplements frequently use the chromium picolinate form which may have slightly higher bioavailability than other forms of chromium (2). Chromium picolinate is chromium bound to picolinic acid, a natural derivative of the amino acid tryptophan which is thought to facilitate chromium absorption (3).

Claimed benefits

Improved body composition, more lean muscle tissue and less fat tissue.

Mode of Action

Chromium combines with a complex of nicotinic acid and the amino acids glycine, cysteine and glutamic acid to form a complex called Glucose Tolerance Factor. This enhances the effect of insulin and increases muscular uptake of nutrients which in turn reduces the available excess nutrients to be stored as fat. The precise mechanism of this effect is not well understood but it is believed that the complex increases the sensitivity of the insulin receptor and increases the number of glucose transporters which translocate to the cell membrane in response to insulin (1), (4).

Effectiveness

Studies carried out on diabetics show that chromium supplementation may have a small positive effective on blood glucose and insulin sensitivity (5), (6), (7), (8).

However in healthy people a multitude of studies have failed to find any benefit or improvement in strength or body composition either in sedentary individuals (9) or combined with various types of exercise programs including resistance training (10), (11), (12), (13), a Navy physical conditioning program (14) and a wrestling training program (15).

Commonly used dosages

Chromium is usually contained in sport supplements in combination with other ingredients, often as part of a fat loss product. Amounts from as low as 8mcg up to 300mcg can be seen.

When sold as a stand alone supplement capsules from 200mcg to 500mcg can be found.

Safety

Chromium is regarded as non-toxic and safe even at high doses. Due to this the US Food and Nutrition Board of the Institute of Medicine has not set a tolerable upper level of intake (1), (4) and neither has the European Food Safety Authority (16). In addition, in the diabetes studies intakes of 1000mcg for up to 4 months have been shown to be safe (17).

However isolated adverse reactions have occurred, mainly with chromium picolinate. There are two reports of kidney damage occurring in people taking chromium picolinate (18), (19) and a single report of liver damage (20).

Previous concerns regarding the genotoxicity (damaging to DNA and therefore potentially cancer causing) of chromium picolonate have been found to be unproven after investigation by health agencies (2), (4).

Interactions

Due to its possible insulin enhancing effects chromium may increase the risk of hypoglycemic episodes in those taking medication for the treatment of diabetes.

Chromium picolinate at doses of 1000mcg has been reported

to decrease the absorption of the thyroid medication levothyroxine by up to 17% so it would be wise to avoid taking the two together (21).

References

1. Chromium. Linus Pauling Institute. [online] at http://lpi.oregonstate.edu/infocenter/minerals/chromiu m/
2. Chromium picolinate, zinc picolinate and zinc picolinate dihydrate added for nutritional purposes in food supplements. European Food Safety Authority. [online] at http://www.efsa.europa.eu/EFSA/efsa_locale-1178620753812_1211902603290.htm
3. Executive Summary Chromium Picolinate. National Toxicology Program. [online] at http://ntp.niehs.nih.gov/index.cfm?objectid=6F5E980E -F1F6-975E-7CA23E823F2CB959
4. Mason P. Dietary Supplements. 3rd ed. London: Pharmaceutical Press; 2007
5. Althuis MD, Jordan NE, Ludington EA, Wittes JT. Glucose and insulin responses to dietary chromium supplements: a meta-analysis. Am J Clin Nutr. 2002;76(1):148-55
6. Broadhurst CL, Domenico P. Clinical studies on chromium picolinate supplementation in diabetes mellitus--a review. Diabetes Technol Ther. 2006;8(6):677-87
7. Fox GN, Sabovic Z. Chromium picolinate supplementation for diabetes mellitus. J Fam Pract. 1998;46(1):83-6
8. Martin J, Wang ZQ, Zhang XH, Wachtel D, Volaufova J. *et al.* Chromium picolinate supplementation attenuates body weight gain and increases insulin sensitivity in subjects with type 2 diabetes. Diabetes Care. 2006;29(8):1826-32

9. Amato P, Morales AJ, Yen SS. Effects of chromium picolinate supplementation on insulin sensitivity, serum lipids, and body composition in healthy, nonobese, older men and women. J Gerontol A Biol Sci Med Sci. 2000;55(5):M260-3

10. Hallmark MA, Reynolds TH, DeSouza CA, Dotson CO, Anderson RA, Rogers MA. Effects of chromium and resistive training on muscle strength and body composition. Med Sci Sports Exerc. 1996;28(1):139-44

11. Lukaski HC, Bolonchuk WW, Siders WA, Milne DB. Chromium supplementation and resistance training: effects on body composition, strength, and trace element status of men. Am J Clin Nutr. 1996;63(6):954-65

12. Hasten DL, Rome EP, Franks BD, Hegsted M. Effects of chromium picolinate on beginning weight training students. Int J Sport Nutr. 1992;2(4):343-50

13. Campbell WW, Joseph LJ, Davey SL, Cyr-Campbell D, Anderson RA, Evans WJ. Effects of resistance training and chromium picolinate on body composition and skeletal muscle in older men. J Appl Physiol. 1999 Jan;86(1):29-39

14. Trent LK, Thieding-Cancel D. Effects of chromium picolinate on body composition. J Sports Med Phys Fitness. 1995;35(4):273-80

15. Walker LS, Bemben MG, Bemben DA, Knehans AW. Chromium picolinate effects on body composition and muscular performance in wrestlers. Med Sci Sports Exerc. 1998;30(12):1730-7

16. Tolerable Upper Intake Levels for Vitamins and Minerals by the Scientific Panel on Dietetic products, nutrition and allergies (NDA) and Scientific Committee on Food (SCF). European Food Safety Authority. [online] at http://www.efsa.europa.eu/EFSA/efsa_locale-1178620753812_1178633962601.htm

17. Anderson RA, Cheng N, Bryden NA, Polansky MM, Cheng N. *et al.* Elevated intakes of supplemental

chromium improve glucose and insulin variables in individuals with type 2 diabetes. Diabetes. 1997;46(11):1786-91

18. Wasser WG, Feldman NS, D'Agati VD. Chronic renal failure after ingestion of over-the-counter chromium picolinate. Ann Intern Med. 1997;126(5):410

19. Wani S, Weskamp C, Marple J, Spry L. Acute tubular necrosis associated with chromium picolinate-containing dietary supplement. Ann Pharmacother. 2006;40(3):563-6. Epub 2006 Feb 21

20. Lança S, Alves A, Vieira AI, Barata J, de Freitas J, de Carvalho A. Chromium-induced toxic hepatitis. Eur J Intern Med. 2002;13(8):518-520.

21. John-Kalarickal J, Pearlman G, Carlson HE. New medications which decrease levothyroxine absorption. Thyroid. 2007;17(8):763-5.

Cissus Quadrangularis

Other names

Asthisamhrta
Hadjod
Hadjora
Harbhanga
Hasjora
Pirandai
Veldt-grape
Vitis quadrangularis
Winged treebine

Star rating

1

What is it?

A woody climbing plant of the Vitaceae family found in many countries but mainly in tropical regions.

Claimed benefits

Anabolic action and improved healing of tendons and ligaments.

Mode of Action

Original research on cissus quadrangulis carried out mainly in India in the 1960's and 1970's discovered that it promoted the healing of fractured bones. This research mentioned that a natural anabolic steroid present in the plant was responsible for this effect which led to claims of it promoting muscle growth and also stimulating the repair of tendons and ligaments.

Effectiveness

More modern research has revealed that the steroid present in cissus quadrangularis is a phytoestrogen which acts on the estrogen receptors in bone. Estrogen has anabolic action in bone by reducing the activity of osteoclasts which are cells which break down bone. Cissus quadrangulis is also believed to increase the uptake of the minerals calcium, sulphur and strontium by the osteoblasts (cells which build up bone) during fracture healing (1), (2).

Clearly an estrogenic steroid will not promote muscular anabolism as is claimed. Nor is there any evidence that this compound or its mechanism of action could have a beneficial effect on tendon or ligament healing.

Commonly used dosages

Cissus quadrangularis is often included as part of a proprietary formulation in commercial sport supplement preparations with the exact quantity of the substance not listed in the ingredients.

When the quantity is listed amounts of 500mg to 1000mg have been seen.

When sold as a stand alone supplement an amount of 750mg is usual.

Safety

No known safety issues.

Interactions

None known.

References

1. Shirwaikar A, Khan S, Malini S. Antiosteoporotic effect of ethanol extract of Cissus quadrangularis Linn. on ovariectomized rat. J Ethnopharmacol. 2003;89(2-3):245-50
2. Deka DK, Lahon LC, Saikia J, Mukit A. Effect of Cissus Quadrangularis in accelerating healing process of experimentally fractured radius-ulna of dog: a preliminary study. Indian J Pharmacol 1994;26: 44 - 45

Citrulline malate

Other names

(2S)-2-amino-5-(carbamoylamino)pentanoic acid; 2-hydroxybutanedioic acid
L-Ornithine, N5-(aminocarbonyl)-, mono(+-)-hydroxybutanedioate
Stimol

Star rating

3

What is it?

A compound formed from citrulline and malate and having the molecular formula $C_{10}H_{19}N_3O_8$. Citrulline is an α-amino acid formed in the urea cycle which takes place in the liver and removes ammonia from the body. Malate is an intermediate compound formed in the Krebs cycle which is a cellular metabolic pathway involved in the chemical conversion of carbohydrates, fats and proteins into energy.

Claimed benefits

Improved aerobic performance, reduction of fatigue and improved recovery from exercise.

Mode of Action

During intense exercise the muscles produce waste products such as ammonia and lactic acid which are removed by the urea and Krebs cycles. If not removed quickly enough these byproducts can accumulate and are believed to play a role in producing muscle fatigue.

Supplementation with citrulline malate which supplies essential compounds for the functioning of the urea and Krebs cycles is believed to improve the efficiency with which these cycles operate and enable the faster removal of waste products hence delaying the onset of fatigue and aiding recovery.

Effectiveness

In vivo animal studies tested rats infected with a toxin to artificially induce muscle fatigue. Rats who were orally supplemented with citrulline malate had increased resistance to fatigue (1), (2).

In humans two studies have indicated a beneficial effect of citrulline malate on aerobic energy production leading to delayed onset of fatigue and enhanced recovery after exercise. In the first, eighteen men complaining of fatigue but with no documented disease were given oral supplementation with 6 g/day of citrulline malate for 15 days and subjected to a finger exercise protocol. Metabolism of the finger muscle was analyzed by 31P magnetic resonance spectroscopy which showed a 34% increase in the rate of aerobic energy production during exercise, and a 20% increase in the rate of phosphocreatine recovery after exercise (3).

In the second study 30 basketball players were split into two equal groups. The first group consumed between 12g and 18g of citrulline malate daily for 13 days. The second group consumed 6g daily. The amount of work each person could do in a cycle ergometer exercise test before their blood lactate concentration reached 4mmol/L (the aerobic-anaerobic threshold) was tested before and after the 13 day period. Statistically significant increases in the aerobic-anaerobic threshold were observed in the first group but not the second group. Additionally, 27% of the people in group 1 were able to achieve a higher maximal workload overall (4).

Commonly used dosages

Citrulline malate is usually included as part of a proprietary formulation in commercial sport supplement preparations with the exact quantity of the substance not listed in the ingredients.

When the amount is listed an amount of 3000mg per serving is commonly seen.

It is also available as a stand alone supplement sold in the form of a powder.

Safety

No known safety issues.

Interactions

None known.

References

1. Goubel F, Vanhoutte C, Allaf O, Verleye M, Gillardin JM. Citrulline malate limits increase in muscle fatigue induced by bacterial endotoxins. Can J Physiol Pharmacol. 1997;75(3):205-7
2. Giannesini B, Izquierdo M, Le Fur Y, Cozzone PJ, Verleye M. *et al*. Beneficial effects of citrulline malate on skeletal muscle function in endotoxemic rat. Eur J Pharmacol. 2009;602(1):143-7. Epub 2008 Nov 17
3. Bendahan D, Mattei JP, Ghattas B, Confort-Gouny S, Le Guern ME, Cozzone PJ. Citrulline/malate promotes

aerobic energy production in human exercising muscle. Br J Sports Med. 2002;36(4):282-9

4. Janeira MA, Maia JR, Santos PJ. Citrulline malate effects on the aerobic-anaerobic threshold and in post exercise blood lactate recovery. Med Sci Sports Exerc 1998; 30(5 supp): abstract 881.

Conjugated Linoleic Acid

Other names

Bovinic acid
Cis-9,trans-11 conjugated linoleic acid
CLA-Triacylglycerol
Rumenic acid
Trans-10,cis-12 conjugated linoleic acid

Star rating

4

What is it?

Conjugated linoleic acid (CLA) is a polyunsaturated fatty acid which occurs naturally in many foods particularly those from ruminant animals such as beef and dairy products. The body cannot synthesize its own CLA.

There are 28 known isomers (different forms) of CLA, however only two forms have been shown to possess biological activities. These are the cis-9, trans-11 and trans-10, cis-12 forms (1). In natural food sources the cis-9, trans-11 isomer predominates by 30–70:1 (2) however CLA supplements are usually produced by processing plant oils such as safflower which results in a product containing high levels of both the cis-9, trans-11 and the trans-10,cis-12 isomers.

Claimed benefits

Improved body composition, less fat and more lean muscle mass.

Mode of Action

Evidence from animal and cell studies suggests that the cis-9, trans-12 isomer is the form responsible for anabolic effects and increases in muscle mass whilst the trans-10, cis-12 isomer is the form which causes increased lipolysis and fat oxidation.

CLA affects enzymes regulating fat metabolism causing reduced fat storage in adipocytes (fat storage cells), and increased mobilization and oxidation of fats for energy. It also seems to reduce adipocyte proliferation and induces apoptosis (cell death) of developing adipocytes (2).

Effectiveness

CLA has been shown to be effective in animal studies and has reduced body fat percentage in animals such as mice, rats and pigs. Mice seem to respond best to CLA with 40%-80% reductions in body fat mass being observed when CLA composed 0.5% of their diet (2). In mice CLA has been shown to decrease fat mass while simultaneously increasing muscle mass (3) (4) (5).

In humans one or two small studies have shown no benefit from CLA supplementation (6). The results of other studies have been underappreciated on the grounds that CLA did not reduce overall bodyweight or BMI even though fat mass was significantly reduced, which strongly indicates a concomitant increase in lean mass.

However as more recent and larger studies have been published using more accurate methods of fat measurement the weight of evidence has shifted squarely in favour of the beneficial effect of CLA on body composition.

For example a year long double blind study looked at 180 healthy but overweight men and women randomized to receive either placebo or 4.5g CLA daily (equivalent to approximately 3.6g of active isomers as a 50:50 mixture of cis-9, trans-11 and trans-10, cis-12 isomers). After 12 months the CLA group had approximately 7-8% less body fat mass than the placebo group (as measured by the accurate dual-energy X-ray absorptiometry method) and approximately 2% more lean body mass (7).

In a follow on study 134 of the original participants in the above study were then given a 4.5g daily dose of CLA (regardless of whether they had originally received CLA or a placebo) for a further 12 months. The individuals originally taking a placebo then had an average reduction in body fat mass of approximately 6%. The people who had already been taking CLA maintained their reduction in body fat mass but did not lose any more (8).

A later double blind, placebo-controlled trial involving 118 people also looked at which body site CLA caused the greatest reduction in fat mass, comparing arms, legs and abdomen. After 6 months supplementation with a similar quantity and type of CLA as used in the studies above body fat mass was significantly reduced by 3.4% after 6 months supplementation with CLA compared with placebo. The reduction in fat mass was located mostly in the legs and women had more loss than men. There was also a significant reduction in the waist/hip ratio (9).

Other smaller studies in obese individuals have shown similar results regarding loss of fat mass (10) (11) and gain in lean body mass (12).

Studies on non-obese healthy exercising humans have also shown a beneficial but small effect of CLA. For example in a randomised double blind study of 76 men and women supplemented with 5g daily of CLA and undertaking resistance training for 14 weeks a statistically significant reduction in fat mass of 4% and an increase in lean body mass of 2.3% was seen. Most of the participants had more than 2 years of resistance training experience and had been training at least two times per week for a minimum of 3 months before involvement in the study (13).

Other studies with exercising individuals have seen similar results (14) (15).

In conclusion CLA supplementation will probably lead to modest reductions in body fat mass and modest increases in lean body mass.

Commonly used dosages

CLA is commonly found in meal replacement formulas and bars in doses from 1000mg to 1500mg.

It is also sold as a stand alone supplement often in capsules of 1000mg containing between 70%-80% CLA.

Safety

CLA did not produce serious adverse effects in the studies

mentioned above when taken for periods up to 24 months.

The most common adverse effects reported were gastrointestinal upset including nausea and diarrhea.

There is some concern that the isolated trans-10,cis-12 isomer of CLA can increase insulin resistance which can be a risk factor for or worsen diabetes or the metabolic syndrome. It is not known if commercial supplements containing mixed isomers have the same effect (16) (17).

Interactions

None known.

References

1. Banni S. Conjugated linoleic acid metabolism. Curr Opin Lipidol. 2002;13(3):261-6
2. Wahle KW, Heys SD, Rotondo D. Conjugated linoleic acids: are they beneficial or detrimental to health? Prog Lipid Res. 2004;43(6):553-87
3. DeLany JP, Blohm F, Truett AA, Scimeca JA, West DB. Conjugated linoleic acid rapidly reduces body fat content in mice without affecting energy intake. Am J Physiol. 1999;276(4 Pt 2):R1172-9
4. West DB, Delany JP, Camet PM, Blohm F, Truett AA *et al*. Effects of conjugated linoleic acid on body fat and energy metabolism in the mouse. Am J Physiol. 1998;275(3 Pt 2):R667-72
5. Park Y, Albright KJ, Liu W, Storkson JM, Cook ME *et al*. Effect of conjugated linoleic acid on body composition in mice. Lipids. 1997;32(8):853-8
6. Zambell KL, Keim NL, Van Loan MD, Gale B, Benito P *et al*. Conjugated linoleic acid supplementation in humans:

effects on body composition and energy expenditure. Lipids. 2000;35(7):777-82

7. Gaullier JM, Halse J, Høye K, Kristiansen K, Fagertun H *et al.* Conjugated linoleic acid supplementation for 1 y reduces body fat mass in healthy overweight humans. Am J Clin Nutr. 2004;79(6):1118-25

8. Gaullier JM, Halse J, Høye K, Kristiansen K, Fagertun H *et al.* Supplementation with conjugated linoleic acid for 24 months is well tolerated by and reduces body fat mass in healthy, overweight humans. J Nutr. 2005;135(4):778-84

9. Gaullier JM, Halse J, Høivik HO, Høye K, Syvertsen C *et al.* Six months supplementation with conjugated linoleic acid induces regional-specific fat mass decreases in overweight and obese. Br J Nutr. 2007 Mar;97(3):550-60

10. Risérus U, Berglund L, Vessby B. Conjugated linoleic acid (CLA) reduced abdominal adipose tissue in obese middle-aged men with signs of the metabolic syndrome: a randomised controlled trial. Int J Obes Relat Metab Disord. 2001;25(8):1129-35

11. Blankson H, Stakkestad JA, Fagertun H, Thom E, Wadstein J *et al.* Conjugated linoleic acid reduces body fat mass in overweight and obese humans. J Nutr. 2000 Dec;130(12):2943-8

12. Steck SE, Chalecki AM, Miller P, Conway J, Austin GL *et al.* Conjugated linoleic acid supplementation for twelve weeks increases lean body mass in obese humans. J Nutr. 2007;137(5):1188-93

13. Pinkoski C, Chilibeck PD, Candow DG, Esliger D, Ewaschuk JB *et al.* The effects of conjugated linoleic acid supplementation during resistance training. Med Sci Sports Exerc. 2006;38(2):339-48

14. Thom E, Wadstein J, Gudmundsen O. Conjugated linoleic acid reduces body fat in healthy exercising humans. J Int Med Res. 2001 Sep-Oct;29(5):392-6

15. Kreider RB, Ferreira MP, Greenwood M, Wilson M, Almada AL. Effects of conjugated linoleic acid supplementation during resistance training on body composition, bone density, strength, and selected hematological markers. J Strength Cond Res. 2002;16(3):325-34
16. Risérus U, Smedman A, Basu S, Vessby B. Metabolic effects of conjugated linoleic acid in humans: the Swedish experience. Am J Clin Nutr. 2004 Jun;79(6 Suppl):1146S-1148S
17. Risérus U, Arner P, Brismar K, Vessby B. Treatment with dietary trans10cis12 conjugated linoleic acid causes isomer-specific insulin resistance in obese men with the metabolic syndrome. Diabetes Care. 2002 Sep;25(9):1516-21

Creatine Monohydrate

Other names

(alpha-Methylguanido)acetic acid
2-[carbamimidoyl(methyl)amino]acetic acid
Creatin
Kreatin
Krebiozon
Methylglycocyamine
N-(Aminoiminomethyl)-N-methylglycine
N-amidinosarcosine
N-methyl-N-guanylglycine
Pyrolysate

Star rating

5

What is it?

An amino acid found mainly in skeletal and cardiac muscle which participates in the transfer of high energy phosphate during the anaerobic phase of muscle contraction. Creatine phosphate transfers its phosphate to adenosine diphosphate (ADP) creating the energy molecule adenosine triphosphate (ATP). Creatine is produced in the liver, pancreas and kidneys from the precursor amino acids arginine, glycine and methionine. The kidneys form guanidinoacetate from arginine and glycine which the liver methylates to form creatine.

About two thirds of muscle creatine is stored as phosphocreatine while a third is stored as free creatine (1). The average diet supplies approximately 1-2g of creatine daily mainly from animal sources such as meat. Minimal amounts are found in plants.

Claimed benefits

Increases lean muscle mass, increases strength, increases high intensity (anaerobic) exercise capacity.

Mode of Action

Creatine supplementation works to increase high intensity exercise capacity by increasing muscle stores of creatine and phosphocreatine which increases the energy available to synthesize ATP and maintain high intensity exercise (1).

Creatine also has three distinct mechanisms by which it increases strength and muscle mass.

Firstly, creatine drives water into muscle fibre cells via osmosis. Creatine loading at a dose of 20g/day for 5 days typically results in a 1-3kg increase in bodyweight due to increased muscle fluid content (2). Evidence exists that the increased muscle fibre volume this produces acts as a stimulus for increased cellular protein synthesis (3).

Secondly, creatine supplementation increases production of the myogenic regulatory factors Myo-D, myogenin, MFR-4, and Myf5 in muscle cells. These regulatory factors increase the adaptive response of muscles to resistance training causing greater muscle hypertrophy than observed with training alone (3).

Thirdly, creatine increases the number of satellite cells and muscle cell myonucei present in muscle fibres. Muscle fibre cells possess several myonuclei which control their function. As muscle fibres increase in size the number of myonuclei required also increases. New myonuclei are produced by adjacent cells called satellite cells. Strength training by itself has been shown to increase the number of satellite cells and the number of new myonuclei produced. However creatine supplementation plus strength training has been proven to increase satellite cell numbers and myonuclei production even more than with training alone producing an even greater hypertrophic response (3).

Effectiveness

Creatine is one of the most intensively studied sports supplements and has several hundred studies confirming its effectiveness. It is accepted by the International Society of Sports Nutrition (ISSN) and the American College of Sports Medicine as an effective ergogenic aid which performs as claimed. The ISSN has stated that creatine is "the most effective nutritional supplement currently available in terms of improving lean body mass and anaerobic capacity" (1) (4).

Creatine has been shown to be effective for increasing muscle creatine stores by varying amounts depending on the individuals initial creatine levels. For individuals with high initial levels such as trained athletes creatine can increase total stores by up to 20%. For people with low initial stores such as sedentary individuals or vegetarians then the increase can be up to 40%. This typically translates into average improvements in performance and strength of 5 - 15%.

These improvements have been observed in a wide variety of disciplines such as cycling, sprinting, weight training, swimming and soccer. In studies of weight training individuals subjects taking creatine typically gain twice as much lean muscle tissue than subjects not taking creatine (1).

It should be pointed out however that approximately 10% of the population are apparent "non-responders" to creatine supplementation. The reasons for this are not well understood but appears to occur in individuals with naturally high initial levels of muscle creatine (3).

Creatine monohydrate is the form of creatine that has been most extensively studied and is most commonly used in sports supplements. Recently various other forms of creatine have begun to be marketed such as creatine phosphate and creatine ethyl ester to name two. However there is no evidence that any of these different formulations are more effective than creatine monohydrate and they are usually more expensive. In addition there is much less safety data for the newer forms of creatine compared to creatine monohydrate (5).

Commonly used dosages

The most commonly used protocol and that followed in the majority of creatine studies is to begin with a loading dose of 20g/day for 5 – 7 days followed by a maintenance dose of 3 – 5g/day. This protocol has been shown to maximally increase muscle creatine stores.

An alternative protocol which omits the loading phase and involves just taking 3 – 5g/day is also effective but muscle creatine stores take longer to reach maximal levels with this method.

Cycling protocols consisting of repeating the loading phase described above every 3 to 4 weeks but without taking any maintenance dose between loading cycles are also reported to be effective at increasing muscle creatine levels (1).

Several recent studies suggest that muscle uptake of creatine is up to 60% greater when the creatine is consumed with a carbohydrate such as dextrose compared to taking creatine alone probably due to the effect of increased insulin levels (1).

Safety

Various anecdotal and media claims have appeared over the years claiming that creatine can cause muscle cramps and dehydration. This has led to recommendations to avoid using creatine when training in hot environments.

There is no scientific evidence for these claims and neither muscle cramps nor dehydration have been reported in any of the many creatine studies. In addition recent studies show that creatine may in fact improve performance in hot and humid conditions by improving hydration and body temperature control and reducing the amount of fluid lost through sweat (6).

There is also a common misconception that creatine use can negatively affect kidney function. In fact several studies have shown that creatine has no effect on either liver or kidney function in healthy individuals and this applies for both young and old subjects even when taking creatine for several months. It would be prudent nevertheless for those with kidney problems to avoid taking creatine (7).

In other studies no long term safety concerns have arisen in groups of people after taking creatine for up to 5 years (1).

Interactions

The interaction between caffeine and creatine is not clear. In one small study of 9 people taking either caffeine with creatine or creatine alone there was no difference in muscle creatine levels when measured. The caffeine plus creatine group however apparently had lower performance in an exercise test (8). On the other hand other studies have found that caffeine and creatine together improve performance (9) (10). Given that the original study found no effect of caffeine on the ability of creatine to increase muscle creatine levels its findings regarding an adverse effect on performance should be viewed with caution.

References

1. Buford TW, Kreider RB, Stout JR, Greenwood M, Campbell B *et al*. International Society of Sports Nutrition position stand: creatine supplementation and exercise. J Int Soc Sports Nutr. 2007;4:6
2. Dalbo VJ, Roberts MD, Stout JR, Kerksick CM. Putting to rest the myth of creatine supplementation leading to

muscle cramps and dehydration. Br J Sports Med. 2008;42(7):567-73. Epub 2008 Jan 9

3. Aagaard P. Making muscles "stronger": exercise, nutrition, drugs. J Musculoskelet Neuronal Interact. 2004;4(2):165-74
4. American Dietetic Association; Dietitians of Canada; American College of Sports Medicine, Rodriguez NR, Di Marco NM, Langley S. American College of Sports Medicine position stand. Nutrition and athletic performance. Med Sci Sports Exerc. 2009;41(3):709-31
5. Jäger R, Purpura M, Shao A, Inoue T, Kreider RB. Analysis of the efficacy, safety, and regulatory status of novel forms of creatine. Amino Acids. 2011 Mar 22. [Epub ahead of print]
6. Dalbo VJ, Roberts MD, Stout JR, Kerksick CM. Putting to rest the myth of creatine supplementation leading to muscle cramps and dehydration. Br J Sports Med. 2008;42(7):567-73. Epub 2008 Jan 9
7. Kim HJ, Kim CK, Carpentier A, Poortmans JR. Studies on the safety of creatine supplementation. Amino Acids. 2011 Mar 12. [Epub ahead of print]
8. Vandenberghe K, Gillis N, Van Leemputte M, Van Hecke P, Vanstapel F, Hespel P. Caffeine counteracts the ergogenic action of muscle creatine loading. J Appl Physiol. 1996;80(2):452-7
9. Doherty M, Smith PM, Davison RC, Hughes MG. Caffeine is ergogenic after supplementation of oral creatine monohydrate. Med Sci Sports Exerc. 2002;34(11):1785-92
10. Lee CL, Lin JC, Cheng CF. Effect of caffeine ingestion after creatine supplementation on intermittent high-intensity sprint performance. Eur J Appl Physiol. 2011 Jan 5. [Epub ahead of print]

Damiana

Other names

Damiana Aphrodisiaca
Damiana de Guerrero
Diffusa aphrodisiaca
Mexican damiana
Mexican holly
Turnera aphrodisiaca
Turnera diffusa
Turnera microphylla
Turnerae diffusae folium
Turnerae Diffusae Herba

Star rating

2

What is it?

A small shrub belonging to the Turneraceae family found throughout Mexico, Central America, South America and the West Indies. It has long been used in traditional medicine throughout the world particularly as an aphrodisiac.

Claimed benefits

Improves libido. Loss of libido can be a side effect experienced on cessation of other anabolic and androgenic substances used by sports people.

Sometimes claimed to increase testosterone levels.

Mode of Action

Unknown.

Damiana was identified in an *in vitro* study (1) as being an aromatase inhibitor. Since the enzyme aromatase converts tesosterone into estrogen, blocking its action would raise testosterone levels and could account for a libido enhancing effect, however the ability of Damiana to do this *in vivo* has not been tested.

Various flavonoids present in Damiana have been identified as having anti aromatase activity, among these flavanone pinocembrin showed the strongest inhibitory activity. Another flavonone present in Damiana called acacetin is structurally analagous to the flavone chrysin (5,7-dihydroxyflavone), present in the blue passion flower (Passiflora caerulea), which is also a known aromatase inhibitor.

Damiana was also reported to have strong affinity for progesterone receptors. Since some progestins have androgenic effects this could be another possible mechanism of action for the libido enhancing effects of Damiana.

Effectiveness

There are no human studies investigating the use of Damiana as a libido enhancer or on its ability to increase testosterone levels.

It has been demonstrated to act as an aphrodisiac by increasing sexual activity in sexually sluggish/impotent male rats, but having no effect on normal male rats (2) (3).

Commonly used dosages

Damiana is commonly included in sport supplements in amounts from 50mg – 100mg along with various other ingredients.

When used alone, traditionally doses are 2 - 4 grams dried leaf three times daily or 2 - 4 mL of liquid extract (4).

When sold as a stand alone supplement Damiana is commonly available in capsules of 400mg – 500mg or as a fluid extract.

Safety

No known safety issues.

Damiana is approved for food use in the USA and Europe (4).

Interactions

Damiana has been shown to have hypoglycemic effects in mice and so may potentiate the effect of diabetes medication (5).

References

1. Zhao J, Dasmahapatra AK, Khan SI, Khan IA. Anti-aromatase activity of the constituents from damiana (Turnera diffusa). J Ethnopharmacol. 2008;120(3):387-93. Epub 2008 Sep 26
2. Arletti R, Benelli A, Cavazzuti E, Scarpetta G, Bertolini A. Stimulating property of Turnera diffusa and Pfaffia paniculata extracts on the sexual-behavior of male rats. Psychopharmacology (Berl). 1999;143(1):15-9

3. Estrada-Reyes R, Ortiz-López P, Gutiérrez-Ortíz J, Martínez-Mota L. Turnera diffusa Wild (Turneraceae) recovers sexual behavior in sexually exhausted males. J Ethnopharmacol. 2009;123(3):423-9. Epub 2009 Mar 31
4. Barnes J, Anderson LA, Phillipson JD. Herbal Medicines. 3rd ed. London: Pharmaceutical Press; 2007
5. Pérez RM, Ocegueda A, Muñoz JL, Avila JG, Morrow WW. A study of the hypoglycemic effect of some Mexican plants. J Ethnopharmacol. 1984 Dec;12(3):253-62

Dandelion

Other names

Cankerwort
Herba Taraxaci
Leontodon taraxacum
Lion's tooth
Pu Gong Ying
Taraxacum dens-leonis
Taraxacum officinale
Taraxacum palustre
Taraxacum vulgare

Star rating

3

What is it?

A flowering plant of the genus Taraxacum in the family Asteraceae which are native to Europe and Asia. It is widely used as a herbal medicine in many cultures.

Claimed benefits

Diuretic.

Mode of Action

Unknown.

Effectiveness

Few studies have been carried out on the diuretic effect of dandelion and those that have have been somewhat contradictory. For example two animal studies on rats failed to find any diuretic effect when they were administered an ethanolic and aqueous root extract of dandelion (1), (2).

However these studies used a root extract whereas another study compared root extract with leaf extract and found leaf extract to possess much greater diuretic activity. In this study administration of leaf extract to male rats at a dose equivalent to 8 g dried herb/kg body weight induced considerable diuresis leading to a 30% loss of body weight (3).

In the only known human study, 17 people were given a high quality fresh leaf hydroethanolic extract of dandelion and monitored over the course of a day. This resulted in a statistically significant increase in both the frequency and volume of urination and in the 5-hour period after ingestion of the extract (3).

Commonly used dosages

Dandelion is commonly included in sport supplements in doses from 100mg to 250mg as part of a weight loss formula containing various ingredients.

It is available as a stand alone supplement in the form of a liquid extract or in the form of capsules usually containing 500mg of dandelion.

Safety

There is an isolated report of a dandelion containing product causing heart arrythmias in one person, however the product also contained bladderwrack, and boldo and it is unknown which of the ingredients (if any) caused this reaction (4).

Interactions

Dandelion may potentiate the effect of other diuretic drugs. Dandelion contains high levels of potassium and so may cause dangerously high potassium levels if taken with potassium sparing diuretics such as spironolactone (6).

References

1. Tita B, Bello U, Faccendini P, Bartolini R, Bolle P. Taraxacum officinale W.: pharmacological effect of ethanol extract. Pharmacol Res 1993;27:23–24.
2. Grases F, Melero G, Costa-Bauz´a A, Prieto R, March J.G. Urolithiasis and phytotherapy. Int Urol Nephrol 1994;26:507–511
3. Rácz-Kotilla E, Rácz G, Solomon A. The action of Taraxacum officinale extracts on the body weight and diuresis of laboratory animals. Planta Med. 1974;26(3):212-7
4. Clare BA, Conroy RS, Spelman K. The diuretic effect in human subjects of an extract of Taraxacum officinale Folium over a single day. J Altern Complement Med. 2009;15(8):929-34
5. Agarwal SC, Crook JR, Pepper CB. Herbal remedies -- how safe are they? A case report of polymorphic

ventricular tachycardia/ventricular fibrillation induced by herbal medication used for obesity. Int J Cardiol 2006;106:260-1.

6. Williams CA, Goldstone F, Greenham J. Flavonoids, cinnamic acids and coumarins from the different tissues and medicinal preparations of Taraxacum officinale. Phytochemistry 1996;42:121-7.

Danshen

Other names

Chinese sage
Dan Shen
Fufang Danshen
Radix Salviae miltiorrhiza
Red sage root
Salvia Miltiorrhiza
Tanshen
Tan-Shen

Star rating

2

What is it?

A perennial flowering plant in the genus Salvia native to Japan and China. The roots are used in traditional Chinese medicine mainly for the treatment of heart conditions and strokes.

Claimed benefits

Aids fat loss and helps prevent weight gain.

Mode of Action

Excess calories are converted by the body into triglycerides and stored as fat. The diacylglycerol acyltransferase (DGAT) enzymes catalyze the final step in triglyceride synthesis by linking an sn-1,2-diacylglycerol with a fatty acyl CoA to form a triacylglycerol, or triglyceride.

Preventing the formation of triglycerides by inhibiting the action of DGAT may therefore help prevent the storage of fat in the body. The roots of Salvia miltiorrhiza contain eighteen compounds called abietane diterpenes (tanshinones) and four of these have been found to inhibit DGAT in rat liver cells *in vitro* (1).

The most potent of these was cryptotanshinone followed closely by 15,16-dihydrotanshinone. The other two tanshinone I and tanshinone IIA only inhibited DGAT very weakly.

Effectiveness

Danshen has not been tested on living animals or humans either in regard to its ability to inhibit DGAT or for its ability to control weight.

Studies involving genetically manipulated mice so they had non functioning DGAT produced mice which had 50% less fat and smaller adipocytes (fat cells) than normal mice. These mice were resistant to weight gain when fed a high fat diet. These mice also had normal muscle mass and there was no adverse effect on blood triglyceride levels suggesting that

DGAT does not play a rate-limiting role in hepatic secretion of triglycerides (2).

In humans it has been found that there is a genetic variation in the efficiency at which DGAT is able to synthesize triglycerides. In a study (3) involving 1322 Turkish people it was found that women who had the genes for a less active form of DGAT had a 6.8% lower BMI, 10% higher HDL cholesterol levels (good cholesterol) and 8% lower diastolic blood pressures than women with more active DGAT. However no differences were seen in men regardless of their DGAT genes.

This indicates that inhibiting DGAT levels in humans might be a useful strategy for controlling weight, however more research is needed to discover what extent sexual and racial differences affect the role played by DGAT in controlling weight. Further research is also needed to confirm whether danshen is in fact able to affect DGAT in humans.

Commonly used dosages

Danshen is usually included as part of a proprietary formulation in commercial sport supplement preparations with the exact quantity of the substance not listed in the ingredients (note: Danshen is usually listed by its scientific name Salvia Miltiorrhiza on sport ingredient labels).

When the amount is listed amounts of 250mg can be seen.

Caution: Many supplements state that the extract is standardized to contain a certain amount of tanshinones (typically 30% - 40%) but do not state which ones so it is assumed it is a mixture of all of them but contains mainly tanshinone I and tanshinone IIA which are the most abundant tanshinones present in Danshen but are also the weakest DGAT inhibitors. However some supplements e.g. Gaspari Nutrition Plasmajet ® specifically state that the extract is standardized for cryptotanshinone which is the most potent DGAT inhibitor.

Danshen is difficult to find as a stand alone supplement.

Safety

No known safety issues.

Interactions

Danshen may increase the effect of warfarin and increase the risk of bleeding. You should avoid using Danshen if you are on warfarin or other drugs which increase the risk of bleeding such aspirin, clopidogrel and heparin (4) (5).

Danshen may interfere with the measurement of digoxin levels and you should avoid taking it if you are on this drug (6).

References

1. Ko JS, Ryu SY, Kim YS, Chung MY, Kang JS *et al.* Inhibitory activity of diacylglycerol acyltransferase by tanshinones from the root of Salvia miltiorrhiza. Arch Pharm Res. 2002;25(4):446-8
2. Chen HC, Farese RV Jr. Inhibition of triglyceride synthesis as a treatment strategy for obesity: lessons from DGAT1-deficient mice. Arterioscler Thromb Vasc Biol. 2005;25(3):482-6. Epub 2004 Nov 29
3. Ludwig EH, Mahley RW, Palaoglu E, Ozbayrakçi S, Balestra ME *et al.* DGAT1 promoter polymorphism associated with alterations in body mass index, high

density lipoprotein levels and blood pressure in Turkish women. Clin Genet. 2002;62(1):68-73

4. Izzo AA, Di Carlo G, Borrelli F, Ernst E. Cardiovascular pharmacotherapy and herbal medicines: the risk of drug interaction. Int J Cardiol. 2005 Jan;98(1):1-14

5. Holbrook AM, Pereira JA, Labiris R, McDonald H, Douketis JD *et al.* Systematic overview of warfarin and its drug and food interactions. Arch Intern Med. 2005;165(10):1095-106

6. Wahed A, Dasgupta A. Positive and negative in vitro interference of Chinese medicine dan shen in serum digoxin measurement. Elimination of interference by monitoring free digoxin concentration. Am J Clin Pathol. 2001;116(3):403-8

DHEA

Other names

(3S,8R,9S,10R,13S,14S)-3-hydroxy-10,13-dimethyl-1,2,3,4,7,8,9,11,12,14,15,16-dodecahydrocyclopenta[a]phenanthren-17-one
(3β)-3-Hydroxyandrost-5-en-17-one
Andrestenol
Androstenolone
Dehydroepiandrosterone
Dehydroisoandrosterone
Diandron
Diandrone
Prasterone
Prestara
Psicosterone
Trans-dehydroandrosterone
Δ5-androsten-3β-ol-17-one

Star rating

2

What is it?

A weakly androgenic hormone mainly produced and secreted by the adrenal glands although it is also produced in small amounts by the testes and ovaries. It circulates in the blood as dehydroepiandrosterone sulfate (DHEA-S) the storage form of DHEA which is converted in target tissues to DHEA. DHEA can then be converted to other hormones, including estrogens and androgens such as testosterone.

Claimed benefits

Improves muscle mass and strength and promotes fat loss.

Mode of Action

By acting as a precursor to testosterone, supplementation with DHEA is theorized to increase circulating levels of this anabolic hormone.

DHEA has also been shown to stimulate insulin like growth factor-1 (IGF-1) which can enhance insulin sensitivity and increase muscle growth (1).

Effectiveness

Few studies have been carried out in relation to DHEA supplementation and increases in strength and muscle mass and those that exist mainly focused on supplementation in older individuals.

One small randomized double-blind placebo-controlled

cross-over trial (2) with 19 subjects (men and women) aged 50 to 65 given 100mg DHEA daily for 6 months found that in men, but not in women, fat body mass decreased approximately 6% and that strength as measured by knee extension and back exercises increased around 15%.

However a much larger and longer double blind placebo controlled study (3) which administered 50mg/day of DHEA to 280 men and women aged 60 to 80 during 12 months found that although serum DHEAS levels were returned to the normal range for young adults (aged 20-50 years) no positive effect was observed either on muscle strength or on muscle and fat mass.

Finally a study (4) involving 19 men with an average age of 23 and undertaking a resistance training program for 8 weeks found no effect on testosterone levels after taking 150mg of DHEA and no effect on strength or muscle mass.

In summary there is little current evidence that DHEA is of value to sports people.

Commonly used dosages

DHEA is usually included as part of a proprietary formulation in commercial sport supplement preparations with the exact quantity of the substance not listed in the ingredients.

It is widely available as a stand alone supplement in doses from 25mg to 100mg with recommended intakes of 50mg to 100mg daily.

Safety

At higher doses DHEA may cause androgenic side effects

such as acne and increased body hair growth.

There is a small theoretical risk that DHEA may increase the risk of prostate, breast and other hormone dependent cancers.

There have been isolated reports of DHEA inducing mania at doses as low as 50mg/day (5) (6).

Interactions

As DHEA can be coverted to estrogen it may reduce the effectivenes of aromatase inhibiting drugs such as letrozole, anastrozole, exemestane and other estrogen receptor antagonist drugs such as tamoxifen (7).

References

1. Casson PR, Santoro N, Elkind-Hirsch K, Carson SA, Hornsby PJ. Postmenopausal dehydroepiandrosterone administration increases free insulin-like growth factor-I and decreases high-density lipoprotein: a six-month trial. Fertil Steril. 1998;70(1):107-10
2. Morales AJ, Haubrich RH, Hwang JY, Asakura H, Yen SS. The effect of six months treatment with a 100 mg daily dose of dehydroepiandrosterone (DHEA) on circulating sex steroids, body composition and muscle strength in age-advanced men and women. Clin Endocrinol (Oxf). 1998;49(4):421-32
3. Percheron G, Hogrel JY, Denot-Ledunois S, Fayet G, Forette F *et al*. Effect of 1-year oral administration of dehydroepiandrosterone to 60- to 80-year-old individuals on muscle function and cross-sectional area: a double-blind placebo-controlled trial. Arch Intern Med. 2003;163(6):720-7

4. Brown GA, Vukovich MD, Sharp RL, Reifenrath TA, Parsons KA *et al.* Effect of oral DHEA on serum testosterone and adaptations to resistance training in young men. J Appl Physiol. 1999;87(6):2274-83
5. Markowitz JS, Carson WH, Jackson CW. Possible dihydroepiandrosterone-induced mania. Biol Psychiatry 1999;45:241-2.
6. Dean CE. Prasterone (DHEA) and mania. Ann Pharmacother 2000;34:1419-22.
7. Calhoun K, Pommier R, Cheek J, Fletcher W, Toth-Fejel S. The effect of high dehydroepiandrosterone sulfate levels on tamoxifen blockade and breast cancer progression. Am J Surg. 2003;185(5):411-5

7-Keto-DHEA

Other names

7-keto Dehydroepiandrosterone
7-oxo-DHEA
7-oxo-dehydroepiandrosterone-3-acetate
7-oxo Dehydroepiandrosterone
3-acetyl-7-oxo-dehydroepiandrosterone
3 beta-acetoxy-androst-5-ene-7,17-dione

Star rating

3

What is it?

A metabolite of DHEA (dehydroepiandrosterone) produced in the body and which is not converted into testosterone or estrogen. Therefore oral supplementation with 7-keto-DHEA does not affect the levels of these hormones in the body (1).

Claimed benefits

Fat loss.

Mode of Action

7-keto-DHEA has been shown to induce the thermogenic (calorie burning) enzymes mitochondrial sn-glycerol-3-phosphate dehydrogenase and cytosolic malic enzyme in the livers of rats which are known to metabolize DHEA in a similar way to humans (1).

There is also some preliminary evidence that 7-keto-DHEA can increase levels of the thyroid hormone triiodothyronine (T3) which is responsible for energy regulation (2) (3).

Effectiveness

Only one small study has has been conducted to assess the fat loss effects of 7-keto-DHEA which gave either a placebo or 7-keto-DHEA 100mg twice a day to 28 women and 2 men for 8 weeks (although 7 people dropped out before the end of the study). They also undertook an exercise program 3 times a week. The 7-keto-DHEA group experienced a –1.8% drop in body fat compared to –0.57% for the placebo group. The 7-keto-DHEA group also experienced a significant increase in T3 levels compared with the placebo group of +17.88 ng/dL compared to +2.75 ng/dL. There were no significant changes in levels of thyroid-stimulating hormone (TSH), thyroxine (T4), testosterone or estrogen.

Commonly used dosages

7-keto-DHEA can be found in commercial sport supplements in amounts from 100mg to 150mg usually together with various other ingredients as part of a proprietary blend.

It is easily obtained as a stand alone supplement in the form of capsules containing from 25mg to 200mg.

Safety

No known safety issues.

Interactions

None known.

References

1. Lardy H, Partridge B, Kneer N, Wei Y. Ergosteroids: induction of thermogenic enzymes in liver of rats treated with steroids derived from dehydroepiandrosterone. Proc Natl Acad Sci U S A. 1995;92(14):6617-9
2. Kalman DS, Colker CM, Swain MA, Torina GC, Shi Q. A Randomized, Double-Blind, Placebo Controlled Study of 3Acetyl-7-Oxo-Dehydroepiandrosterone in Healthy Overweight Adults. Curr Ther Res Clin Exp 2000;61(7):435-442
3. Colker C, Torina G, Swain M, Kalman D. Double-Blind, Placebo-Controlled, Randomized Clinical Trial Evaluating the Effects of Exercise Plus 3-Acetyl-7-oxodehydroepiandrosterone on Body Composition and the Endocrine System in Overweight Adults. Abstract published in Journal of Exercise Physiology online, Volume 2 Number 4 October 1999.

DIM - Diindolylmethane

Other names

3-(*1H*-Indol-3-ylmethyl)-*1H*-indole
3,3'-Methylenebis-*1H*-indole
3,3'-Diindolylmethane

Star rating

4

What is it?

Cruciferous vegetables such as cabbage, cauliflower, broccoli, and brussels sprouts contain indole-3-glucosinolate (glucobrassicin). On consumption the enzyme myrosinase is released from the plants, which cleaves indole-3-glucosinolate to release indole-3-carbinol (I3C). In the stomach I3C degrades to a reactive indolinium ion intermediate which reacts with I3C or other reactive indolinium ions to form the oligomer DIM (1).

Claimed benefits

Increases testosterone levels
Regulates estrogen metabolism (increases ratio of weak form to strong form)
Promotes fat loss

Mode of Action

In the body endogenous estrogen is metabolized by cytochrome P450 enzymes to either 16alpha-hydroxyestrone (16OHE1) or 2-hydroxyestrone (2OHE1). The 2OHE1 metabolite shows weak estrogenic activity and is commonly referred to as the "good" estrogen. 16OHE1 has strong estrogenic activity (2).

In clinical trials oral supplementation with both I3C and DIM has been shown to increase the ratio of 2OHE1 to 16OHE1 (3), (4), (5), (6). This is achieved via the induction of metabolizing cytochrome P450 enzymes (P450-1A1 and P450-1A2), which facilitate the metabolization of estrogen to 2OHE1 (2).

The resulting reduced level of estrogenic activity can be postulated to have two effects;

- A reduction in bodyfat since estrogen has been implicated in fat storage (7), (8), (9).

- An increase in testosterone levels since a reduction in estrogenic activity would result in less negative feedback on LH (luteinizing hormone) release from the pituitary gland and hence more LH output. LH stimulates the Leydig cells in the testes to produce testosterone (10).

In addition to this mode of action DIM may also act as an estrogen receptor antagonist reducing the ability of estrogen to bind to its receptor (11), (12).

It is frequently claimed by supplement manufacturers that 2OHE1 can "release" testosterone from SHBG and thus increase levels of free testosterone. There is absolutely no evidence for this claim. However the increased level of 2OHE1 may cause a reduction in the level of SHBG formed since estrogen induces SHBG production in the liver (13).

Effectiveness

The ability of DIM to alter estrogen metabolism has been

demonstrated by the studies cited above. However no data is available showing effectiveness for increasing testosterone levels or fat loss.

Commonly used dosages

Usually used at doses of 100mg – 200mg/day. In the study showing that oral DIM supplementation increased the ratio of 2OHE1 the subjects took 108mg/day (6).

Safety

No known safety issues.

Interactions

None known.

However there is some evidence that DIM can increase the activity of the enzyme CYP1A2 (14) and could therefore decrease serum concentrations of medications metabolized by CYP1A2 e.g. propranolol, clozapine, haloperidol (14).

References

1. Diindolylmethane (DIM) Information Resource Center [online] at http://www.diindolylmethane.org/
2. Douglas C. Hall, M.D. Nutritional Influence on Estrogen Metabolism by Applied Nutritional Science Reports, 2001 (article) available online at http://www.cabecahealth.com/PDF%20files/NutrInflue ncesEstrogen.pdf
3. Bradlow HL, Michnovicz JJ, Halper M, Miller DG, Wong GY, Osborne MP. Long-term responses of women to indole-3-carbinol or a high fiber diet. Cancer Epidemiol Biomarkers Prev. 1994;3(7):591-595.

4. McAlindon TE, Gulin J, Chen T, Klug T, Lahita R, Nuite M. Indole-3-carbinol in women with SLE: effect on estrogen metabolism and disease activity. Lupus. 2001;10(11):779-783.
5. Michnovicz JJ. Increased estrogen 2-hydroxylation in obese women using oral indole-3-carbinol. Int J Obes Relat Metab Disord. 1998;22(3):227-229.
6. Dalessandri KM, Firestone GL, Fitch MD, Bradlow HL, Bjeldanes LF. Pilot study: effect of 3,3'-diindolylmethane supplements on urinary hormone metabolites in postmenopausal women with a history of early-stage breast cancer. Nutr Cancer. 2004;50(2):161-167.
7. O'Sullivan AJ, Hoffman DM, Ho KK. Estrogen, lipid oxidation, and body fat. N Engl J Med. 1995;333(10):669-70.
8. O'Sullivan AJ, Martin A, Brown MA. Efficient Fat Storage in Premenopausal Women and in Early Pregnancy: A Role for Estrogen. J. Clin. Endocrinol. Metab. 2001;86: 4951-4956
9. Leung KC, Johannsson G, Leong GM, Ho KKY. Estrogen Regulation of Growth Hormone Action. Endocr. Rev. 2004;25: 693-721
10. Vanderschueren D, Bouillon R. Estrogen deficiency in men is a challenge for both the hypothalamus and pituitary. J Clin Endocrinol Metab. 2000;85(9):3024-6.
11. Chang YC, Riby J, Chang GH, Peng BC, Firestone G, Bjeldanes LF. Cytostatic and antiestrogenic effects of 2-(indol-3-ylmethyl)-3,3'-diindolylmethane, a major in vivo product of dietary indole-3-carbinol. Biochem Pharmacol. 1999;58(5):825-34.
12. Riby JE, Chang GH, Firestone GL, Bjeldanes LF. Ligand-independent activation of estrogen receptor function by 3, 3'-diindolylmethane in human breast cancer cells. Biochem Pharmacol. 2000;60(2):167-77.
13. Loukovaara M, Carson M, Adlercreutz H. Regulation of production and secretion of sex hormone-binding

globulin in HepG2 cell cultures by hormones and growth factors. J Clin Endocrinol Metab. 1995;80(1):160-4.

14. Lake BG, Tredger JM, Renwick AB, Barton PT, Price RJ. 3,3'-Diindolylmethane induces CYP1A2 in cultured precision-cut human liver slices. Xenobiotica. 1998;28(8):803-811.

Dodder

Other names

Chinese Dodder
Cuscuta
Cuscuta chinensis
Cuscuta epithymum
Cuscutae
Devil's guts
Devil's hair
Dodder seed
Goldthread
Hailweed
Scaldweed
Semen Cuscutae
Strangleweed

Star rating

2

What is it?

A genus of parasitic plants found throughout the temperate and tropical regions of the world. Formerly placed in the family Cuscutaceae but now recognised as belonging to the family Convolvulaceae.

Claimed benefits

Increased muscle mass through raised levels of testosterone.

Mode of Action

Various flavanoids have been isolated from dodder of which the five principal ones are quercetin 3-O-beta-D-galactoside-7-O-beta-D-glucoside, quercetin 3-O-beta-D-apiofuranosyl-(1-->2)-beta-D-galactoside, hyperoside, quercetin and kaempferol (1).

These flavanoids are believed to be the active ingredients in dodder which have been shown to increase testosterone levels *in vivo* in rats when given at a dose of 300 mg/kg per day. The presumed mechanism of action being increased luteinizing hormone (LH) production by the pituitary gland since LH levels and pituitary weight also increased. Luteinizing hormone stimulates the Leydig's cells in the testes to produce testosterone (2) (3).

Effectiveness

The ability of dodder to produce increased levels of testosterone or increases in muscle mass in humans has not been tested.

Commonly used dosages

Dodder is usually included as part of a proprietary formulation in commercial sport supplement preparations with the exact quantity of the substance not listed in the ingredients.

It is virtually impossible to find dodder as a stand alone supplement.

Safety

No known safety issues.

Interactions

None known.

References

1. Ye M, Li Y, Yan Y, Liu H, Ji X. Determination of flavonoids in Semen Cuscutae by RP-HPLC. J Pharm Biomed Anal. 2002;28(3-4):621-8
2. Qin DN, She BR, She YC, Wang JH. Effects of flavonoids from Semen Cuscutae on the reproductive system in male rats. Asian J Androl. 2000;2(2):99-102
3. Wang J, Wang M, Ou Y, Wu Q. [Effects of flavonoids from semen Cuscutae on changes of beta-EP in hypothalamuses and FSH and LH in anterior pituitaries in female rats exposed to psychologic stress] Zhong Yao Cai. 2002;25(12):886-8

Ecdysteroids

Other names

11,20-dihydroxyecdysone
20 Beta-Hydroxyecdysterone
20E
20-hydroxyecdysone
Ecdisten
Ecdisteron
Ecdysone
Ecdysterone
Ectysterone
Isoinokosterone
Phytoecdysone
Phytoecdysteroid
Turkesteron
Turkesterone

Star rating

3

What is it?

Ecdysteroids are insect steroid hormones which regulate moulting and reproduction. They have also been discovered occurring naturally in approximately 6% of plant species where they are believed to act as a natural insecticide to defend against insect attack.

Various different ecdysteroids have been identified. The first ecdysteroid isolated in 1954 was ecdysone. The most abundantly occuring ecdysteroid is 20-hydroxyecdysone (also called 20E) which occurs in many plants including spinach and the herb Rhaponticum carthamoides from which many commercial ecdysteroids are extracted. Rhaponticum carthamoides is also a source of turkesterone (also called 11,20-dihydroxyecdysone) which is reported to be the most potent ecdysterone for promoting protein synthesis (1). Turkesterone is also found in Ajuga turkestanica (2).

Over 300 ecdysteroids have been identified which are recorded in an online database at http://ecdybase.org

Claimed benefits

Anabolic action and promote protein synthesis.

Mode of Action

The mechanism of action of ecdysteroids in mammals is currently unknown. Their structure is quite different from mammalian steroids and so it is surmised that they do not interact with mammalian steroid receptors or steroid metabolising enzymes (3). Instead, they may influence signal transduction pathways via membrane bound receptors in a manner similar to anabolic steroids (4).

Effectiveness

Interest in the anabolic properties of ecdysteroids began in the 1960's when it was reported that they were able to stimulate protein synthesis in mouse liver, heart and muscles (1).

Growth promoting and body weight increasing effects have been seen when ecdysteroids are fed to rats, pigs, sheep and quail. For example in pigs doses of 0.2 - 0.4 mg/kg/ per day resulted in better nitrogen retention and average body weight improvements of 112–116% compared to controls (1).

Japanese quail fed 100mg /kg of 20-hydroxyecdysone increased in mass 115% (5).

20-hydroxyecdysone increased muscle fibre size in rats and additionally increased the myonuclear number in the fibres suggesting the activation of satellite cells which control muscle growth (6).

Russian research from the 1980's also showed that ecdysteroids improved physical performance in animal forced exercise tests in a similar fashion to the anabolic steroid methandrostenolone (dianabol) (1).

In their study Wilborn CD *et al.* (7) discuss the results of a Russian study composed of 78 highly trained male and female athletes which showed that ecdysterone and protein intake caused a 6 - 7% increase in lean muscle tissue and a 10% reduction in fat in just 10 days. A second Russian study discussed also showed increased muscle mass and reduced fat mass after ecdysteroid supplementation. Unfortunately Wilborn *et al.* do not discuss the dosing protocols used by the Russians and the original research is no longer available.

Wilborn CD *et al.* do not report similar results from their study. In their randomized double blind placebo controlled trial 11 resistance training males were given 30mg of 20-hydroxyecdysone for 8 weeks. No improvements in training volume, body mass or composition or anabolic/catabolic status were seen. This study can be criticised however on the grounds that the dose of 20-hydroxyecdysone used was equivalent to only 0.36mg/kg of bodyweight per subject which is far below the effective dose reported in other ecdysteroid studies. Most of the animal studies for example used a dose of 5mg/kg, nearly 14x more.

Commonly used dosages

Ecdysteroids are usually included as part of a proprietary formulation in commercial sport supplement preparations with the exact quantity of the substance not listed in the ingredients.

Few ecdysteroids are available as stand alone supplements but there are some ecdysterone stand alone supplements available usually in low doses of around 15mg. I have seen some brands offering much higher amounts for lower prices which tends to suggest there is some variation in the quality or purity of the products being offered.

Recommended doses of these commercial products tends to be around 30mg/day. As noted above the doses used in the majority of the studies has been 5mg/kg which would be equivalent to 350mg/day for a 70kg person.

Human elimination of ecdysteroids is quite rapid. The effective half time of elimination is 4 hours for ecdysterone and 9 hours for 20-hydroxyecdysone so splitting consumption evenly throughout the day would be required to maintain plasma levels elevated (1).

Safety

No known safety issues. The toxicity of ecdysteroids in mammals is low, the LD50 of 20-hydroxyecdysone is >9g/kg in mice when consumed orally. Ecdysteroids and their metabolites are excreted in the urine and faeces.

In addition ecdysteroids appear to exhibit various beneficial health effects including lowering blood sugar and cholesterol, improving liver, kidney, heart and lung function and improving the immune system and having anti-oxidant properties.

Ecdysteroids have no androgenic or estrogenic effects and do not affect blood pressure (1).

Interactions

None known.

References

1. Lafont R, Dinan L. Practical uses for ecdysteroids in mammals including humans: an update. J Insect Sci. 2003;3:7
2. Ecdybase, Turkesterone [online] at http://ecdybase.org/index.php?&action=browse&row=4 33
3. Dinan L, Lafont R. Effects and applications of arthropod steroid hormones (ecdysteroids) in mammals. J Endocrinol. 2006;191(1):1-8
4. Báthori M, Tóth N, Hunyadi A, Márki A, Zádor E. Phytoecdysteroids and anabolic-androgenic steroids-- structure and effects on humans. Curr Med Chem. 2008;15(1):75-91
5. Sláma K, Koudela K, Tenora J, Mathová A. Insect hormones in vertebrates: anabolic effects of 20-hydroxyecdysone in Japanese quail. Experientia. 1996;52(7):702-6
6. Tóth N, Szabó A, Kacsala P, Héger J, Zádor E. 20-Hydroxyecdysone increases fiber size in a muscle-specific fashion in rat. Phytomedicine. 2008;15(9):691-8. Epub 2008 Jun 26
7. Wilborn CD, Taylor LW, Campbell BI, Kerksick C, Rasmussen CJ *et al.* Effects of methoxyisoflavone, ecdysterone, and sulfo-polysaccharide supplementation

on training adaptations in resistance-trained males. J Int Soc Sports Nutr. 2006;3:19-27

Eurycoma Longifolia

Other names

Longifolia jack
Longjack
Malaysian Ginseng
Pasak bumi
Payong ali
Penawar bias
Penawar pahit
Tongkat ali
Tongkat baginda

Star rating

2

What is it?

A shrub/tree in the family Simaroubaceae, native to Indonesia and Malaysia. Traditionally used as a folk medicine to cure impotence and increase fertility and libido. Also used for anti-malarial and anti-pyretic properties.

Claimed benefits

Increased levels of testosterone.

Mode of Action

Usually claimed to stimulate the pituitary to release more luteinizing hormone which in turn stimulates the testes to produce more testosterone.

Effectiveness

The most often cited evidence for an effect on testosterone production by Eurycoma longifolia are comments attributed to a Chinese researcher (1) however it has not been possible to confirm these comments or their validity since the research was not published.

Several studies confirm that Eurycoma longifolia increases libido, sexual interest and frequency of erections in rats and mice (2), (3), (4), (5) but this has not been shown in humans.

It was not demonstrated that these increases in libido are due to an increase in testosterone or that Eurycoma longifolia has any affect on luteinizing hormone.

Two studies indicate that Eurycoma longifolia may have an anabolic action. In one it increased the size of levator ani muscles in rats (6) but no mode of action was proposed. In another very small study it produced increases in lean body mass and strength in 7 men (7).

In a 2005 article (not a study) in Nature Medicine (8) a Malaysian biotechnology company reported having identified a 4.3 kilodalton protein constituent of Eurycoma longifolia which was reported to increase testosterone production. However the article states that the US patent office rejected the company's application.

Commonly used dosages

In the human study reported above the subjects received 100mg/day of a soluble extract. Common doses in commercial preparations are 1500 mg/day to 6000 mg/day.

Safety

No known safety issues.

Interactions

None known.

References

1. Lie-Chwen Lin (National Research Institute of Chinese Medicine, Shih-Pai, Taipei 112, Taiwan, R.O.C.) and Chen-Yuan Peng, Hsing-Shun Wang, Kuo-Wu Lee, and Paulus S. Wang (all of the Department of Physiology, National Yang-Ming University, Shih-Pai, Taipei 112, Taiwan, R.O.C.) in a scientific study into the Chemical Constituents of Eurycoma longifolia.
2. Ang HH, Ikeda S, Gan EK. Evaluation of the potency activity of aphrodisiac in Eurycoma longifolia Jack. Phytother Res 2000;15:435-6
3. Ang HH, Sim MK. Eurycoma longifolia Jack enhances libido in sexually experienced male rats. Exp Anim 1997;46:287-90.
4. Ang HH, Cheang HS, Yusof AP. Effects of Eurycoma longifolia Jack (Tongkat Ali) on the initiation of sexual performance of inexperienced castrated male rats. Exp Anim 2000;49:35-8.
5. Ang HH, Lee KL, Kiyoshi M. Eurycoma longifolia Jack enhances sexual motivation in middle-aged male mice. J Basic Clin Physiol Pharmacol. 2003;14(3):301-8.

6. Ang HH, Cheang HS. Effects of Eurycoma longifolia jack on laevator ani muscle in both uncastrated and testosterone-stimulated castrated intact male rats. Arch Pharm Res 2001;24:437-40.
7. Hamzah S, Yusof A. The Ergogenic Effects of Eurycoma Longifolia Jack: A Pilot Study. Br. J. Sports Med. 2003; 37:464-70.
8. Cyranoski D. Malaysian researchers bet big on home-grown Viagra. [News] Nature Medicine. 2005;11(9):912

Evodiamine

Other names

8,13,13b,14-Tetrahydro-14-methylindolo[2',3':3,4]pyrido[2,1-b]quinazolin-5(7H)-one
Evodia
Evodia Lepta
Evodia officinalis
Evodia rutaecarpa
Evodia rutaecarpa Bentham
Evodiae
Wu-chu-yu

Star rating

2

What is it?

A quinozole alkaloid component of the dried, unripe fruit of Evodia rutaecarpa Bentham (Rutaceae) which belongs to a genus of tropical trees. It has the molecular formula $C_{19}H_{17}N_3O$.

Claimed benefits

Fat loss.
Increased energy.

Mode of Action

Evodiamine may increase the sensation of fullness after eating and delay the return of feelings of hunger since it has been seen to delay the emptying of food from the stomach and gastrointestinal transit in studies on rats (1).

Like capsaicin (see separate entry) evodiamine is a vanilloid receptor agonist (2) though it lacks any hot or pungent taste. Evodiamine therefore mimics the thermogenic effect of capsaicin by both enhancing body heat production and increasing heat loss (3) which therefore increases the rate at which calories are burned by the body. This was seen to lead to a loss of fat mass and reduction in bodyweight when evodiamine was fed to rats.

The stimulation of vanilloid receptors also causes an increase in the heart rate and force of cardiac contraction (4) (5).

Like capsaicin, evodiamine also appears to be able to increase the secretion of catecholamines (stimulatory hormones such as adrenaline and noradrenaline) from the adrenal gland (*in vitro* study on cow adrenal cells) (6).

Finally, *in vitro* studies on mice and human cells suggest evodiamine can prevent fat precursor cells from developing into mature adipocytes (fat cells) (7) (8).

Effectiveness

There are no human studies on evodiamine to evaluate either

its thermogenic effect or potential as an aid to fat loss.

It should be noted that one of the studies mentioned above (2) stated that evodiamine was 3 to 19 fold less potent than capsaicin at stimulating the vanilloid receptor. It is unknown if this means that evodiamine would reduce the effect of capsaicin by competing with it for the receptor if they were both taken together and so it would seem wise that these two ingredients should not be combined in a single supplement until more is known about the interaction. (See also note below under interactions regarding evodiamine and caffeine.)

Commonly used dosages

Evodiamine can be found in commercial sport supplements in amounts varying from 5mg to 70mg, usually in combination with a variety of other ingredients.

The lack of human studies makes it hard to evaluate these doses.

Evodiamine is not usually sold as a stand alone supplement.

Safety

No known safety issues.

Interactions

Evodiamine itself has no known interactions. However rutaecarpine another quinozole alkaloid found in Evodia rutaecarpa is known to have anti-platelet properties (9) (10) which means it could increase the risk of bruising and bleeding in people taking drugs such as aspirin, clopidogrel, heparin and warfarin. Due to the similarity in structure between evodiamine and rutaecarpine it is possible that evodiamine also has anti-platelet effects and so should be avoided by anyone taking these drugs.

Similarly, both rutaecarpine alone and a herbal preparation of Evodia rutaecarpa have been found to significantly decrease blood concentrations of caffeine by 64% and 71% when fed to rats at doses of 25mg/kg and 1g/kg (11). This is probably due to rutaecarpine inducing the liver enzyme CYP1A2 which is the enzyme responsible for the metabolism of caffeine. Inducing CYP1A2 therefore speeds up the removal of caffeine from the body.

Due to the similarity in structure between the two quinozole alkaloids rutaecarpine and evodiamine it is possible that evodiamine also alters the metabolism of caffeine in this way. It therefore seems sensible to recommend that evodiamine should not be included in sport supplements which also contain caffeine as a major active ingredient until more is known about these interactions.

References

1. Wu CL, Hung CR, Chang FY, Lin LC, Pau KY, Wang PS. Effects of evodiamine on gastrointestinal motility in male rats. Eur J Pharmacol. 2002;457(2-3):169-76
2. Pearce LV, Petukhov PA, Szabo T, Kedei N, Bizik F *et al.* Evodiamine functions as an agonist for the vanilloid receptor TRPV1. Org Biomol Chem. 2004;2(16):2281-6. Epub 2004 Jul 27
3. Kobayashi Y, Nakano Y, Kizaki M, Hoshikuma K, Yokoo Y, Kamiya T. Capsaicin-like anti-obese activities of evodiamine from fruits of Evodia rutaecarpa, a vanilloid receptor agonist. Planta Med. 2001;67(7):628-33
4. Shoji N, Umeyama A, Takemoto T, Kajiwara A, Ohizumi Y. Isolation of evodiamine, a powerful cardiotonic

principle, from Evodia rutaecarpa Bentham (Rutaceae). J Pharm Sci. 1986;75(6):612-3

5. Kobayashi Y, Hoshikuma K, Nakano Y, Yokoo Y, Kamiya T. The positive inotropic and chronotropic effects of evodiamine and rutaecarpine, indoloquinazoline alkaloids isolated from the fruits of Evodia rutaecarpa, on the guinea-pig isolated right atria: possible involvement of vanilloid receptors. Planta Med. 2001 Apr;67(3):244-8

6. Yoshizumi M, Houchi H, Ishimura Y, Hirose M, Kitagawa T *et al*. Effect of evodiamine on catecholamine secretion from bovine adrenal medulla. J Med Invest. 1997;44(1-2):79-82

7. Wang T, Wang Y, Kontani Y, Kobayashi Y, Sato Y *et al*. Evodiamine improves diet-induced obesity in a uncoupling protein-1-independent manner: involvement of antiadipogenic mechanism and extracellularly regulated kinase/mitogen-activated protein kinase signaling. Endocrinology. 2008;149(1):358-66. Epub 2007 Sep 20

8. Hu YS, Fahmy H, Zjawiony JK, Davies GE. Inhibitory effect and transcriptional impact of berberine and evodiamine on human white preadipocyte differentiation. Fitoterapia. 2009 Sep 29. [Epub ahead of print]

9. Sheu JR, Kan YC, Hung WC, Su CH, Lin CH *et al*. The antiplatelet activity of rutaecarpine, an alkaloid isolated from Evodia rutaecarpa, is mediated through inhibition of phospholipase C. Thromb Res. 1998;92(2):53-64

10. Sheu JR, Hung WC, Lee YM, Yen MH. Mechanism of inhibition of platelet aggregation by rutaecarpine, an alkaloid isolated from Evodia rutaecarpa. Eur J Pharmacol. 1996;318(2-3):469-75.

11. Tsai TH, Chang CH, Lin LC. Effects of Evodia rutaecarpa and rutaecarpine on the pharmacokinetics of caffeine in rats. Planta Med. 2005;71(7):640-5

Flaxseed Oil

Other names

alpha-Linolenate
alpha-Linolenic acid
alpha-Lnn
Flax seed oil
Linolenate
Linolenic acid
Linum crepitans
Linum humile
Linus usitatissimum
n-3 Fatty Acid
Omega-3 Fatty Acid

Star rating

3

What is it?

The oil extracted from the seeds of the plant *Linus usitatissimum* (Genus *Linum*, family Linaceae) which grows virtually worldwide. It contains approximately 70% of polyunsaturated fatty acids of which around 58% are the omega 3 fatty acid alpha-linolenic acid (ALNA). This makes flaxseed oil one of the richest food sources of ALNA (1).

The remaining fatty acid content of the oil is the omega 6 fatty acid linoleic acid (LA). Both LA and ALNA are essential fatty acids, that is they cannot be synthesized by the body and must be consumed in the diet.

The other main omega 3 fatty acids are eicosopentaenoic acid (EPA) and docosahexaenoic acid (DHA) both found in cold water fish like salmon, mackerel, and tuna. The body is able to convert ALNA into EPA and DHA.

Claimed benefits

Reduces accumulation of body fat.

Mode of Action

An excess intake of calories is the major factor contributing to obesity and the consumption of fats is one the major factors contributing to excessive calorie intake. However there is increasing evidence that the type of fat consumed can play a significant role in the tendency to accumulate fat in addition to just the amount of calories consumed.

Contrary to popular belief as adults gain weight the number of adipocytes (fat cells) that are present increase in number as well as increase in size. In other words they exhibit hyperplasia as well as hypertrophy. This is due to the fact that although mature adipocytes do not divide, a pool of pre-adipocyte cells exist which can be recruited to differentiate into mature adipocytes in response to the consumption of dietary fat. However different types of fat affect these pre-adipocytes in different ways. Some types of fats cause pre-adipocytes to develop into mature adipocytes more readily than other types of fats. In this regard LA appears to stimulate the formation of adipocytes while ALNA appears to inhibit their formation.

LA is converted in the body into another omega 6 fatty acid called arachidonic acid (ARA) which is itself converted into prostacyclin by the action of the cyclo-oxygenase (COX) enzyme system. Prostacyclin then signals pre-adipocytes to develop into mature adipocytes. Omega 3 fatty acids such as ALNA appear to inhibit this process by interfering with the

COX system and thus reduce the production of prostacyclin (2).

Effectiveness

The beneficial effect of increasing the proportion of ALNA in the diet has been demonstrated in several animal studies. For example pups from mice fed an LA-rich diet were 40% heavier and had an increased fat mass compared with mice fed a balanced LA/ALNA diet, a difference in body weight that was maintained into adulthood (3).

Similarly in a study on rats fed diets containing the same number of calories but differing in the proportion LA and ALNA they contained, the rats fed the high ALNA diet gained less weight and less body fat than rats fed a higher proportion of LA (4).

In humans the effects of LA and ALNA on body weight and fat gain have been inferred indirectly. For example a relationship was found between higher levels of ARA and obesity in mediterranean children (5) while in another study 400 elderly men were split into two groups with one group receiving a normal diet while the other group received a diet containing a similar number of calories but with the fats composed almost entirely of LA. At the end of 5 years the LA group had an average body weight 5% higher than the normal diet group (6).

It has been calculated that over the last few decades the amount of LA being consumed in the typical Western diet has been increasing while the ALNA content has been falling (2) which could partly explain the increase in obesity seen over that time.

However all this does not mean that taking ALNA

supplements is justified at the present time. First of all the evidence indicates that the LA/ALNA ratio is important when the calories consumed are the same. So simply taking ALNA supplements which add calories without a corresponding reduction in the amount of LA consumed is unlikely to yield benefit in terms of body compostion.

Secondly there is currently much debate about whether the other health benefits attributed to ALNA such as protection against cardiovascular disease etc. can be explained by its conversion in the body to the other omega 3 fatty acids EPA and DHA or whether it has its own independent effect.

As regards reducing body fat accumulation via reducing prostacyclin formation by inhibiting the activity of the COX enzyme system both EPA and DHA from fish oil do this more effectively than ALNA (with EPA being the most effective) (2). It would therefore seem sensible to recommend that if dietary changes were to be made to increase the amount of omega 3 fatty acids consumed this be done by eating more EPA and DHA containing fish rather than consuming flaxseed oil.

Commonly used dosages

Flaxseed oil is commonly included in weight loss supplements and meal replacement type products in amount from 500mg to 1000mg.

It can also be bought as a stand alone supplement.

As mentioned above it is the ratio of omega 6 to omega 3 fats which is more important than simply adding in another type of fat. Current Western diets contain an omega 6/omega 3 ratio of approximately 15/1 whereas research indicates that the optimal ratio is around 4/1 which would have many health benefits particularly reduced cardiovascular risk (7).

Safety

No known safety issues.

Interactions

There is some evidence that flaxseed oil can increase bleeding time and so may increase the risk of bleeding in people taking antiplatelet drugs such as aspirin, clopidogrel or anticogulant drugs like warfarin. People on these kinds of drugs should avoid flaxseed oil (8).

References

1. Cunnane SC, Ganguli S, Menard C, Liede AC, Hamadeh MJ *et al*. High alpha-linolenic acid flaxseed (Linum usitatissimum): some nutritional properties in humans. Br J Nutr. 1993;69(2):443-53
2. Ailhaud G, Guesnet P, Cunnane SC. An emerging risk factor for obesity: does disequilibrium of polyunsaturated fatty acid metabolism contribute to excessive adipose tissue development? Br J Nutr. 2008;100(3):461-70. Epub 2008 Feb 28.
3. Massiera F, Saint-Marc P, Seydoux J, Murata T, Kobayashi T *et al*. Arachidonic acid and prostacyclin signaling promote adipose tissue development: a human health concern? J Lipid Res. 2003;44(2):271-9. Epub 2002 Nov 4
4. Korotkova M, Gabrielsson BG, Holmäng A, Larsson BM, Hanson LA, Strandvik B. Gender-related long-term effects in adult rats by perinatal dietary ratio of n-6/n-3 fatty acids. Am J Physiol Regul Integr Comp Physiol. 2005;288(3):R575-9

5. Savva SC, Chadjigeorgiou C, Hatzis C, Kyriakakis M, Tsimbinos G *et al*. Association of adipose tissue arachidonic acid content with BMI and overweight status in children from Cyprus and Crete. Br J Nutr. 2004;91(4):643-9
6. Dayton S, Hashimoto S, Dixon W, Pearce ML. Composition of lipids in human serum and adipose tissue during prolonged feeding of a diet high in unsaturated fat. J Lipid Res. 1966;7(1):103-11
7. Simopoulos AP. The importance of the ratio of omega-6/omega-3 essential fatty acids. Biomed Pharmacother. 2002;56(8):365-79
8. Nordström DC, Honkanen VE, Nasu Y, Antila E, Friman C, Konttinen YT. Alpha-linolenic acid in the treatment of rheumatoid arthritis. A double-blind, placebo-controlled and randomized study: flaxseed vs. safflower seed. Rheumatol Int. 1995;14(6):231-4

Forskolin

Other names

17beta-acetoxy-8,13-epoxy-1alpha,6beta,9alpha-
trihydroxylabd-14-en-11-one
[(3R,4aR,5S,6S,6aS,10S,10aR,10bS)-3-ethenyl-6,10,10b-
trihydroxy-3,4a,7,
7,10a-pentamethyl-1-oxo-5,6,6a,8,9,10-hexahydro-2H-
benzo[f]chromen-5-yl]
acetate
Adehl
Boforsin
Coleonol
Coleus
Coleus barbatus
Coleus Forskohlii
Colforsin
Colforsina
Colforsine
Colforsinum
Forskholin
HL-362
L-75-1362B
Ocufors
Plectranthus barbatus

Star rating

3

What is it?

Forskolin is a labdane diterpene the major active compound
extracted from the roots of the plant Coleus Forskohlii, a

member of the mint family (Lamiaceae) and which grows in subtropical climates such as India (1).

Claimed benefits

Fat loss.

Mode of Action

In mammals stored fat is used for energy by its hydrolysis to free fatty acids and glycerol. Fat burning hormones such as nor-epinephrine (nor-adrenaline) bind to adrenergic receptors which in turn activate the guanine nucleotide regulatory subunit of the enzyme adenylate cyclase which activates cAMP (cyclic adenosine monophosphate) which is a signalling molecule. When cAMP is produced it causes the production of the enzyme Hormone Sensitive Lipase which is the enzyme which begins the hydrolysis of fat for energy.

Forskolin seems able to directly activate adenylate cyclase, by-passing the adrenergic receptors, and hence increases levels of cAMP and activates Hormone Sensitive Lipase (2) (3).

Since it is the activation of adrenergic receptors which are responsible for effects like shaking, nervousness, increased blood pressure etc. Forskolin does not produce these side effects common to some other fat burning supplements such as ephedrine.

In addition, there is some evidence that Forskolin can stimulate thyroid function by mimicking the action of thyroid stimulating hormone (TSH) and by enhancing its effects in the thyroid (4) (5).

Effectiveness

The mechanism of action of Forskolin as a lipolytic agent is well established and Forskolin is frequently used as a research substance when a lipolytic agent is needed. It has been demonstrated as a lipolytic in *in vitro* tests on both animal cells (1) (2) (3) and human cells (6) (7). In animal cells it has been seen to have similar lipolytic effectiveness as nor-epinephrine (2).

Unfortunately there are few *in vivo* experiments of its use as a weight loss supplement.

In two very small trials Forskolin appeared to be effective at reducing fat when applied topically to the thigh. In both trials a group of 6 women applied topical Forskolin 5 times a week to one thigh and a placebo to the other, both trials reported increased fat loss in the thigh treated with Forskolin after 4 and 6 weeks.

A few other studies have been conducted on the oral intake of Forskolin but virtually all have been funded by one supplement manufacturer and only one of them has been published in a scientific journal. In this published study which was a randomized, double-blind, placebo-controlled study, 30 obese males were randomized to take either 250 mg of 10% Forskolin extract twice a day for a 12-week period or a placebo. Fat mass was measured using the very accurate DXA scan technique.

After 12 weeks the Forskolin group showed a statistically significant decease in body fat percent of approximately 4% while the placebo group showed no change. There was also a trend towards an increase in lean body mass although his did not quite reach statistical significance (8).

However in another randomized double blind placebo controlled study 23 women also took either 250 mg of 10% Forskolin extract twice a day for a 12-week period or a placebo. On this occasion no statistically significant effect of Forskolin on fat was observed, however the trial was poorly designed since of the 23 participants only 7 took Forskolin while 12 took the placebo which would have made it difficult for any differences to reach statistical significance (9).

Commonly used dosages

Forskolin is usually included in sport supplements together with various other ingredients, usually as part of a fat loss formula.

There seems to be quite a wide variation in the amount of Coleus Forskohlii root included in sport supplements with amounts from 50mg to 150mg being seen. There is also a wide variation in the quality of the extract used with some being standardized for only 10% Forskolin while others state they are standardized for up to 40% Forskolin.

Coleus Forskohlii can also be purchased as a stand-alone supplement in capsules from 100mg to 250mg. These stand-alone products seem to be mainly standardized at 10% Forskolin content.

As mentioned above, in the study demonstrating fat loss, 250mg standardized for 10% Forskolin was taken twice daily.

Safety

No known safety issues.

Interactions

Forskolin has vasodilatory and cardiac inotropic effects. It may theoretically interfere with blood pressure medication or heart medication. It should be avoided by anyone taking these classes of medicines (10).

Additionally, Forskolin can inhibit platelet aggregation and may theoretically increase the risk of bleeding, you should not take Forskolin if you are on warfarin or other drugs which increase the risk of bleeding such aspirin, clopidogrel and heparin (11).

References

1. Ammon HP, Müller AB. Forskolin: from an ayurvedic remedy to a modern agent. Planta Med. 1985;51(6):473-7
2. Morimoto C, Kameda K, Tsujita T, Okuda H. Relationships between lipolysis induced by various lipolytic agents and hormone-sensitive lipase in rat fat cells. J Lipid Res. 2001;42(1):120-7
3. Seamon KB, Daly JW. Forskolin: a unique diterpene activator of cyclic AMP-generating systems. J Cyclic Nucleotide Res. 1981;7(4):201-24
4. van Sande J, Cochaux P, Dumont JE. Forskolin stimulates adenylate cyclase and iodine metabolism in thyroid. FEBS Lett. 1982;150(1):137-41
5. Haye B, Aublin JL, Champion S, Lambert B, Jacquemin C. Chronic and acute effects of forskolin on isolated thyroid cell metabolism. Mol Cell Endocrinol. 1985 Nov;43(1):41-50
6. Löfgren P, Hoffstedt J, Rydén M, Thörne A, Holm C *et al.* Major gender differences in the lipolytic capacity of abdominal subcutaneous fat cells in obesity observed before and after long-term weight reduction. J Clin Endocrinol Metab. 2002;87(2):764-71

7. Imbeault P, Tremblay A, Després J, Mauriège P. beta-adrenoceptor-stimulated lipolysis of subcutaneous abdominal adipocytes as a determinant of fat oxidation in obese men. Eur J Clin Invest. 2000;30(4):290-6
8. Godard MP, Johnson BA, Richmond SR. Body composition and hormonal adaptations associated with forskolin consumption in overweight and obese men. Obes Res. 2005;13(8):1335-43
9. Henderson S, Magu B, Rasmussen C, Lancaster S, Kerksick C *et al.* Effects of coleus forskohlii supplementation on body composition and hematological profiles in mildly overweight women. J Int Soc Sports Nutr. 2005;2:54-62
10. Baumann G, Felix S, Sattelberger U, Klein G. Cardiovascular effects of forskolin (HL 362) in patients with idiopathic congestive cardiomyopathy--a comparative study with dobutamine and sodium nitroprusside. J Cardiovasc Pharmacol. 1990;16(1):93-100
11. Christenson JT, Thulesius O, Nazzal MM. The effect of forskolin on blood flow, platelet metabolism, aggregation and ATP release. Vasa. 1995;24(1):56-61

Geranamine

Other names

1,3-Dimethylamylamine
1,3-Dimethylamylamine HCL
1,3-Dimethylpentylamine
2-Amino-4-methylhexane
2-hexanamine, 4-methyl-
2-Hexanamine, 4-methyl- (9CI)
4-Methyl-2-hexanamine
4-Methylhexan-2-amine
Dimethylamylamine
DMAA
Forthane
Geranium
Methylhexaneamine
Pentylamine, 1,3-dimethyl-

Star rating

1

What is it?

A substance present naturally in the geranium plant (Pelargonium graveolens) a plant indigenous to South Africa. Oil extracted from the plant (used for its scent in the perfume industry) contains 0.7% of geranamine. The oil is also approved for use as a food additive (1).

Geranamine has also been produced synthetically, it was patented in 1944 by the drug company Eli Lilly for use as a nasal decongestant (2).

Claimed benefits

A stimulant and used for weight loss.

Mode of Action

Very little reliable information exists regarding geranamine. It appears to be structurally similar to amphetamines and gives a false positive for amphetamine in drug tests (3). The original Eli Lilly patent reported that geranamine has negligible effects on the central nervous system and is less stimulating than drugs such as ephedrine or amphetamine. However typical sympathetic nervous system effects have been reported such as tremor, nervousness and insomnia (1).

Effectiveness

No known data.

Commonly used dosages

Geranamine is usually included as part of a proprietary formulation in commercial sport supplement preparations with the exact quantity of the substance not listed in the ingredients.

Safety

The Eli Lilly patent claimed that geranamine is relatively non-toxic and safe for oral use although it does not say at what doses.

Geranamine has been used as a recreational "party drug" and there is one case of a 21-year-old male who suffered a cerebral haemorrhage (bleeding in the brain) after taking two pills containing geranamine (4).

The LD50 in mice (the dose of a drug which kills 50% of the animals it is given to) is reported to be 185mg/kg (5).

Interactions

No reliable data available. Given that geranamine is reported to be a stimulant it seems wise to avoid taking it with other stimulant drugs. People with high blood pressure or heart problems should also avoid stimulant drugs.

References

1. Thevis M. Mass Spectrometry in Sports Drug Testing: Characterization of Prohibited Substances and Doping Control Analytical Assays. New Jersey: John Wiley & Sons Inc; 2010
2. European Patent Office. Aminoalkanes. [online] at http://v3.espacenet.com/publicationDetails/originalDoc ument?CC=US&NR=2350318A&KC=A&FT=D&date=19 440530&DB=&locale=
3. Vorce SP, Holler JM, Cawrse BM, Magluilo J Jr. Dimethylamylamine: a drug causing positive immunoassay results for amphetamines. J Anal Toxicol. 2011;35(3):183-7
4. Gee P, Jackson S, Easton J. Another bitter pill: a case of toxicity from DMAA party pills. N Z Med J. 2010;123(1327):124-7
5. United States National Library of Medicine. ChemIDplus Advanced. Methylhexaneamine [online] at http://chem.sis.nlm.nih.gov/chemidplus/ProxyServlet?o bjectHandle=DBMaint&actionHandle=default&nextPage =jsp/chemidheavy/ResultScreen.jsp&ROW_NUM=0&T XTSUPERLISTID=0000105419

Glucuronolactone

Other names

(2R)-2-[(2S,3R,4S)-3,4-dihydroxy-5-oxooxolan-2-yl]-2-
hydroxyacetaldehyde
D-glucofuranurono-6,3-lactone
D-Glucuronic acid γ-lactone
D-Glucuronolactone
Dicurone
Glucoxy
Glucurolactona
Glucurolactone
Glucuron
Glucurone
Glucuronosan
Gluronsan
Guronsan

Star rating

3

What is it?

Glucuronolactone is a metabolite of glucose which is formed
naturally in the human body. Under normal conditions, it is
in equilibrium with glucuronic acid, its immediate precursor,
so the two compounds exist in equal quantities and can be
inter-converted.

Glucuronolactone is also found naturally in a small number
of foods, of which wine is the richest source (up to 20mg/l).
The average adult consumption of glucuronolactone from
food is between 1.2 and 2.3 mg/day. Glucuronolactone

consumed in food is metabolised and excreted as glucaric acid, xylitol and L-xylulose (1).

Claimed benefits

Glucuronolactone is commonly found in energy drinks such as Red Bull® and is often claimed to increase endurance and improve reaction times, concentration and mental alertness.

It is also sometimes claimed to have hepatoprotective (liver protective) properties. It is listed in the Merck Index as a "detoxicant" (2).

Mode of Action

Research carried out by Japanese researchers in the 1960's on both rats and humans suggests that glucuronolactone delays the onset of fatigue by preventing exercised induced reductions in the level of glucuronic acid in the body. Glucuronic acid appears able to detoxify harmful metabolic by-products of exercise. Although the exact mechanism by which it does this is uncertain.

Glucuronolactone was also shown to prevent drops in levels of blood sugar and hepatic glycogen during exercise (3) (4).

I was unable to find any evidence in the scientific literature regarding the hepatoprotective properties of glucuronolactone.

Effectiveness

Most of the human research on the effectiveness of glucuronoactone has unfortunately involved the testing of energy drinks containing various ingredients together, usually caffeine, taurine and glucuronolactone. It is therefore impossible to know which compound in the drink is responsible for the perceived effects and to assess the efficacy of glucuronolactone in isolation.

Having said this, there are several human studies showing that energy drinks containing combinations of these ingredients can improve attention, reaction speed and both aerobic and anaerobic performance (5) (6) (7).

For example one double-blind, randomized, placebo-controlled study involving 12 subjects showed that the energy drink Red Bull ® was able to improve times in a one hour cycling time trial by 4.7% when consumed 40 minutes before exercise (8).

For information regarding the effectiveness of glucuronolactone alone we have to return the Japanese studies from the 1960's mentioned above (3) (4).

These studies may also allow us to separate the effects of glucuronolactone from other ingredients such as caffeine. For example, in repeated running tests on rats, these studies mention that while stimulants such as caffeine and amphetamine were only able to increase the time of the first run to exhaustion, glucuronolactone was also able to prolong the second and third running times when the rat was made to run again.

In further tests involving rats being made to swim until exhaustion, and then being made to swim again, glucuronolactone was again able to significantly prolong the second and third swimming times by up to 25% compared to placebo. Importantly, rats given glucuronolactone also performed better than rats given glucose, fructose or glycogen.

Glucuronolactone was also better at increasing blood sugar and hepatic glycogen during exercise than glucose, fructose or glycogen.

In humans the ability of glucuronolactone supplementation to prevent falls in the level of glucaronic acid in the body during exercise was measured. As stated above glucaronic acid prevents the onset of fatigue by detoxifying metabolic by-products of exercise. A group of 6 rowers had the level of glucaronic acid in their blood and urine measured over several days of rowing practice both before and after glucuronolactone supplementation. After receiving the glucuronolactone, blood levels of glucuronic acid increased over 3 times and urine levels more than doubled. These results suggest a significantly lower level of fatigue after taking glucuronolactone, although unfortunately actual rowing performance was not measured in this study.

Commonly used dosages

One 250ml can of Red Bull® contains 600mg of glucuronolactone, 1000mg of taurine and 80mg of caffeine (8). Participants in the cycling study cited above who showed a 4.7% improvement in their cycling times consumed two cans.

The rowers in the Japanese study who tripled their blood levels of glucaronic acid were given 6 grams a day.

Glucuronolactone can be purchased as a stand alone supplement either as a powder or in capsules, typically containing 500mg.

Safety

One study has been found which reports a link between an

energy drink containing glucuronolactone and transient increases in platelet aggregation and decreases in endothelial function, which are a risk factor for myocardial infarction (heart attack) and stroke. However it is unknown if glucuronolactone was responsible for this effect (9).

Another study (10) found no evidence of adverse effect on cardiovascular or renal function in healthy young people from the consumption of a glucuronolactone containing energy drink (Red Bull®). The same study noted that it had the beneficial effect of ameliorating changes in blood pressure during stressful experiences and increased the participants' pain tolerance.

Interactions

None known.

References

1. Opinion on Caffeine, Taurine and D-Glucurono-γ-Lactone as constituents of so-called "energy" drinks. European Commission. Jan 21, 1999. [online] at http://ec.europa.eu/food/fs/sc/scf/out22_en.html
2. The Merck Index 14th Ed. New Jersey, Merck & Co. Inc. 2006.
3. Tamura S, Tsutsumi S, Tomizawa S, Suguru N, Kizu K, Ito H, *et al*. Metabolism of Glucuronic Acid in Fatigue Due to Physical Exercise. Jpn J Pharmacol 1966;16.2: 138-56.
4. Tamura S, Tsutsumi S, Ito H, Nakai K, Masuda M. Effects of Glucuronolactone and the Other Carbohydrates on the Biochemical Changes Produced in the Living Body of Rats by Hard Exercise. Jpn J Pharmacol 1968;18.1: 30-8.

5. van den Eynde F, van Baelen PC, Portzky M, Audenaert K. The effects of energy drinks on cognitive performance. Tijdschr Psychiatr. 2008;50(5):273-81

6. Reyner LA, Horne JA. Efficacy of a 'functional energy drink' in counteracting driver sleepiness. Physiol Behav. 2002;75(3):331-5

7. Alford C, Cox H, Wescott R. The effects of red bull energy drink on human performance and mood. Amino Acids. 2001;21(2):139-50

8. Ivy JL, Kammer L, Ding Z, Wang B, Bernard JR, Liao YH, Hwang J. Improved cycling time-trial performance after ingestion of a caffeine energy drink. Int J Sport Nutr Exerc Metab. 2009;19(1):61-78

9. Worthley MI, Prabhu A, De Sciscio P, Schultz C, Sanders P, Willoughby SR. Detrimental effects of energy drink consumption on platelet and endothelial function. Am J Med. 2010;123(2):184-7

10. Ragsdale FR, Gronli TD, Batool N, Haight N, Mehaffey A, *et al.* Effect of Red Bull energy drink on cardiovascular and renal function. Amino Acids. 2010;38(4):1193-200. Epub 2009 Aug 4

Glutamine

Other names

(2S)-2,5-diamino-5-oxopentanoic acid
2-Amino-4-carbamoylbutanoic acid
2-aminoglutaramic acid
Gln
glutamic acid 5-amide
Levoglutamide
Levoglutamine
L-glutamine
Q

Star rating

2

What is it?

A non essential amino acid which is the most abundant amino acid in the human body. It is produced from glutamate and ammonia by many body tissues including muscles, kidney, heart, liver and lungs.

Claimed benefits

Improves recovery from intense exercise.

Anabolic action.

Prevents post exercise immune system suppression and protects against minor infections.

Mode of Action

Improved recovery via increased post-exercise glycogen re-synthesis and increased protein synthesis.

Anabolic action via increased protein synthesis.

Immune system support by preventing post exercise falls in glutamine levels which is used for energy by immune system cells.

Effectiveness

The first question to answer regarding glutamine supplementation is whether it can be effectively absorbed in an oral form. There is a trend in sport supplements to promote protein bound or peptide bonded forms of glutamine which are claimed to have a much higher bioavailability than simple free form L-glutamine.

It is true that most L-glutamine consumed orally never makes it to the blood stream since it is used by the intestines for energy. In fact approximately 65% of orally consumed glutamine is used by the intestines in this way (1). However this means that 35% is absorbed and in fact blood levels of glutamine rise in an almost linear dose dependent fashion as more glutamine is consumed (2).

Secondly several studies have demonstrated that protein or peptide bonded forms of glutamine are either absorbed no better than free form L-glutamine (3) or are in fact absorbed worse (4). Therefore if one chose to supplement with glutamine the free form L-glutamine type would be the sensible choice.

Now we will address the question of whether increasing

blood levels of glutamine can increase muscle protein synthesis.

Several *in vitro* studies conducted on animal cells have shown that increasing intramuscular concentrations of glutamine have an anabolic effect by preventing protein breakdown and increasing protein synthesis (5) (6) (7).

In humans the picture is not quite as clear. Most of the studies involving glutamine supplementation in humans have involved acutely unwell patients in catabolic states suffering from trauma, burns or post-surgery. In these groups of people glutamine supplementation has been shown to be beneficial in improving outcomes and in particular in helping to enhance net protein synthesis in skeletal muscle (8) (9).

However in these groups of people glutamine supplementation should be viewed as correction of a glutamine deficiency rather than true supplementation since after severe stress glutamine is mobilized from the muscle to provide energy and hence muscle levels are reduced. Under these circumstances glutamine becomes a conditionally essential amino acid since the body uses more than it can produce.

Since this is not the case with healthy individuals these studies are not really helpful in assessing the benefit of glutamine to healthy athletes. Those few studies which have been conducted on healthy individuals are equivocal.

One *in vivo* study (10) on five healthy male volunteers found no benefit on protein synthesis measured in arm and leg tissues from oral glutamine intake. In fact the glutamine seemed to compete unfavourably with the uptake of other key amino acids such as methionine and phenylalanine, which are indispensable in muscles for protein synthesis. Another study (11) involving seven men and four women did find a small increase in protein synthesis, although this study is difficult to interpret since the glutamine was provided in a mixture of amino acids mimicking the amino acid structure of muscle of which glutamine was only a part (40g of amino acids containing 5.8g glutamine).

Regarding the next claim, that of the ability of glutamine to increase muscle glycogen concentrations after exercise the results of studies have again been disappointing. Glutamine is no more effective at replenishing glycogen than glucose nor does it have any added benefit when added to glucose. In fact re-feeding with carbohydrates can replenish glycogen to three times the level of glutamine, and no doubt three times more cheaply (12) (13).

Finally we will consider the claim that glutamine can prevent an exercise induced immuno-suppression and help athletes avoid developing minor infections post exercise.

It is commonly believed that individuals undertaking intense exercise are more prone to catching minor infections, particularly infections of the upper respiratory tract such as colds and sore throats. Work done in the 1990's by Castell *et al.* at Oxford University in the UK monitored the rates of infections in runners and rowers and found that the rates of such infections were higher in individuals undertaking more intense exercise (14).

Glutamine is important for the function of immune cells such as lymphocytes and macrophages which use it as an energy source. The glutamine is supplied by muscle cells which contain the largest store of glutamine in the body (15).

Different types of exercise may cause a reduction in plasma

glutamine levels. Although different studies have shown varying results, on balance both prolonged exercise such as marathon running and short duration high intensity exercise such as resistance training lower plasma glutamine levels by up to 20% for between 2-4 hours (15).

On this basis a study by Castell *et al.* in the 1990's gave 151 athletes either a 5g glutamine drink at 30 minutes and 2 hours after exercise or a placebo. 81% of the athletes taking the glutamine reported no infections in the following 7 days while only 49% of those taking a placebo reported no infections (14).

However, subsequent studies cast doubt on this result and indicate that low glutamine levels are not responsible for the post exercise suppression of the immune system. Data from Castell *et al.* and other studies have shown that plasma glutamine concentration decreases by a similar degree in both glutamine and placebo-supplemented groups and that there is no significant difference in glutamine levels between subjects who do or do not develop infections (15).

Furthermore, studies which have objectively examined immune system function by measuring parameters such as lymphocyte trafficking, NK and lymphokine-activated killer cell activities and T cell proliferation have found that glutamine supplementation does not prevent post exercise immune system suppression (16) (17).

In summary the evidence that a post exercise reduction in plasma glutamine is due to increased consumption by immune cells and that glutamine supplementation can prevent the temporary immuno-suppression that occurs is weak.

In light of the above discussion it is not surprising to find that the (few) studies of glutamine on exercise performance have failed to find any benefit either on immediate performance when consumed immediately prior to exercise or over a period of 6 weeks.

One study of 6 resistance trained men consuming approximately 23g of glutamine one hour prior to exercise did not find any improvement in their performance on the leg press or bench press compared to placebo (18).

Another study composed of 31 young adults failed to find any improvement in strength or lean body mass after undergoing 6 weeks of glutamine supplementation and a resistance training program (19).

In conclusion there is little evidence for the use of glutamine for any of its claimed benefits to athletes or sports people.

Commonly used dosages

Glutamine is most commonly sold as a powder with recommendations to consume 5 – 20g per day.

Some timed release formulations of glutamine are also sold. In order to maintain a high plasma glutamine concentration it is necessary to supplement with glutamine every 30 minutes (15), so there is some logic to this. However the amounts released are likely to be too low to have any benefit.

The evidence shows that less glutamine is used by the intestines as the amount consumed increases. When 1.5g is consumed the amount used by the intestines is as high as 75% compared with 55% when doses of 9g are consumed (11).

This indicates that timed release formulas are likely to be far less effective at increasing blood levels of glutamine than consuming a large amount of standard glutamine in one go.

Safety

No adverse effects have been seen from short term supplementation with doses up to 60g/day in hospital patients (20).

There has been a report of two individuals developing mania after consuming 2g and 4g a day of glutamine (21). The condition disappeared on cessation of glutamine intake.

Interactions

None known

References

1. Haisch M, Fukagawa NK, Matthews DE. Oxidation of glutamine by the splanchnic bed in humans. Am J Physiol Endocrinol Metab. 2000;278(4):E593-602
2. Déchelotte P, Darmaun D, Rongier M, Hecketsweiler B, Rigal O, Desjeux JF. Absorption and metabolic effects of enterally administered glutamine in humans. Am J Physiol. 1991;260(5 Pt 1):G677-82
3. Boza JJ, Dangin M, Moënnoz D, Montigon F, Vuichoud J *et al.* Free and protein-bound glutamine have identical splanchnic extraction in healthy human volunteers. Am J Physiol Gastrointest Liver Physiol. 2001l;281(1):G267-74
4. Boza JJ, Maire J, Bovetto L, Ballèvre O. Plasma glutamine response to enteral administration of glutamine in human volunteers (free glutamine versus protein-bound glutamine). Nutrition. 2000;16(11-12):1037-42

5. MacLennan PA, Brown RA, Rennie MJ. A positive relationship between protein synthetic rate and intracellular glutamine concentration in perfused rat skeletal muscle. FEBS Lett. 1987 May 4;215(1):187-91
6. MacLennan PA, Smith K, Weryk B, Watt PW, Rennie MJ. Inhibition of protein breakdown by glutamine in perfused rat skeletal muscle. FEBS Lett. 1988 Sep 12;237(1-2):133-6
7. Wu GY, Thompson JR. The effect of glutamine on protein turnover in chick skeletal muscle in vitro. Biochem J. 1990;265(2):593-8
8. Wilmore DW. The effect of glutamine supplementation in patients following elective surgery and accidental injury. J Nutr. 2001;131(9 Suppl):2543S-9S; discussion 2550S-1S
9. Boelens PG, Nijveldt RJ, Houdijk AP, Meijer S, van Leeuwen PA. Glutamine alimentation in catabolic state. J Nutr. 2001;131(9 Suppl):2569S-77S; discussion 2590S
10. Svanberg E, Möller-Loswick AC, Matthews DE, Körner U, Lundholm K. The effect of glutamine on protein balance and amino acid flux across arm and leg tissues in healthy volunteers. Clin Physiol. 2001;21(4):478-89
11. Mittendorfer B, Volpi E, Wolfe RR. Whole body and skeletal muscle glutamine metabolism in healthy subjects. Am J Physiol Endocrinol Metab. 2001;280(2):E323-33
12. Bowtell JL, Gelly K, Jackman ML, Patel A, Simeoni M, Rennie MJ. Effect of oral glutamine on whole body carbohydrate storage during recovery from exhaustive exercise. J Appl Physiol. 1999;86(6):1770-7
13. Rennie MJ, Bowtell JL, Bruce M, Khogali SE. Interaction between glutamine availability and metabolism of glycogen, tricarboxylic acid cycle intermediates and glutathione. J Nutr. 2001;131(9 Suppl):2488S-90S; discussion 2496S-7S

14. Castell LM, Poortmans JR, Newsholme EA. Does glutamine have a role in reducing infections in athletes? Eur J Appl Physiol Occup Physiol. 1996;73(5):488-90
15. Hiscock N, Pedersen BK. Exercise-induced immunodepression- plasma glutamine is not the link. J Appl Physiol. 2002 Sep;93(3):813-22
16. Krzywkowski K, Petersen EW, Ostrowski K, Kristensen JH, Boza J, Pedersen BK. Effect of glutamine supplementation on exercise-induced changes in lymphocyte function. Am J Physiol Cell Physiol. 2001;281(4):C1259-65
17. Rohde T, MacLean DA, Pedersen BK. Effect of glutamine supplementation on changes in the immune system induced by repeated exercise. Med Sci Sports Exerc. 1998;30(6):856-62
18. Antonio J, Sanders MS, Kalman D, Woodgate D, Street C. The effects of high-dose glutamine ingestion on weightlifting performance. J Strength Cond Res. 2002;16(1):157-60
19. Candow DG, Chilibeck PD, Burke DG, Davison KS, Smith-Palmer T. Effect of glutamine supplementation combined with resistance training in young adults. Eur J Appl Physiol. 2001;86(2):142-9
20. Garlick PJ. Assessment of the safety of glutamine and other amino acids. J Nutr. 2001 Sep;131(9 Suppl):2556S-61S
21. Mebane AH. L-Glutamine and mania. Am J Psychiatry 1984;141(10):1302-3

Glycyrrhetinic acid

Other names

(3β,20β)-20-Carboxy-11-oxo-30-norolean-12-en-3-yl 2-O-β-D-glucopyranuronosyl-α-D-glucopyranosiduronic acid
10-hydroxy-2,4a,6a,6b,9,9,12a-heptamethyl-13-oxo-3,4,5,6,6a,7,8,8a,10,
11,12,14b-dodecahydro-1H-picene-2-carboxylic acid
3-Glycyrrhetinic acid
Beta-Glycyrrhetic acid
Beta-Glycyrrhetinic acid
Beta-Glycyrrhetinic acid
Biosone
Enoxolone
Glyccyrhetic acid
Glycyrrhetic acid
Glycyrrhetin
Glycyrrhizic Acid
Glycyrrhizinic acid
Uralenic acid

Star rating

3

What is it?

A triterpine saponin extracted from the root of the herb licorice (Glycyrrhiza glabra).

Carbenoxolone is a synthetic analogue of glycyrrhetinic acid.

Claimed benefits

Fat loss.

Mode of Action

Glycyrrhetinic acid inhibits the activity of the enzyme Type I 11β-hydroxysteroid dehydrogenase (11β-HSD1). This enzyme converts inactive cortisone to active cortisol. Cortisol is involved in the deposition and accumulation of fat tissue. 11β-HSD1 activity has been demonstrated in the subcutaneous fat tissue of humans *in vivo*. By blocking its activity the action of cortisol and hence fat deposition is reduced (1) (2) (3).

There is also evidence (human *in vivo* study) that inhibiting 11β-HSD1 activity with carbenoxolone can increase hepatic insulin sensitivity and decrease glucose production (4).

Effectiveness

There are no studies specifically testing oral supplementation with glycyrrhetinic acid for fat loss, however the effect of consumption of licorice has been tested (5). In 15 people who consumed 3.5g a day for 2 months of a commercial licorice preparation, statistically significant reductions in fat mass as, measured by skinfold thickness and bioelectrical impedance analysis, were observed of between 1 to 3 kilos. However the subjects suffered the side effect of having the hormones renin and aldosterone suppressed, which led to increased water retention and no overall loss in weight.

This is a recognized side effect of excess licorice consumption known as apparent mineralocorticoid excess syndrome which is caused by inhibition of the Type II form of 11β-HSD by glycyrrhetinic acid and which can lead to a dangerous hypokalemic hypertension.

Of more interest is a study carried out using topical

application of a 2.5% glycyrrhetinic acid cream (6). This double blind randomized study was interesting in that although the number of subjects in the study was small (18 women between 18 and 33 years old) the study was well designed in that in addition to having a control group who used a placebo cream, the participants only applied the cream to one thigh. Hence any reduction in fat could be compared to the other thigh, so the subjects also acted as their own control. The fat measurements were also carried out using an accurate ultrasound method in addition to taking measurements of thigh circumference, which further adds credibility to the results.

After applying the cream for a month, statistically significant reductions in the thickness of the superficial subcutaneous fat layer as measured by ultrasound were seen, both in relation to the untreated leg and to the placebo control group. Statistically significant reductions in thigh circumference were also seen. The mean reduction in fat thickness was 2.1 mm and the mean reduction in thigh circumference was 3mm. Although these reductions seem quite small it should be pointed out that the subjects were not dieting or exercising during the study.

No changes were observed in plasma renin, aldosterone, cortisol or blood pressure which indicates that there was minimal or no systemic absorption of the glycyrrhetinic acid. Also, no changes in the thickness of the deep subcutaneous layer of fat were observed, which also indicates the inability of topical glycyrrhetinic acid to be absorbed past the superficial fat layer. Topical application of glycyrrhetinic acid therefore seems very unlikely to produce the apparent mineralocorticoid excess syndrome seen with oral consumption.

Commonly used dosages

Glycyrrhetinic acid can be found in some topical fat loss supplements currently sold however it is usually included as part of a proprietary blend of several ingredients with the exact quantities not disclosed. I have not seen it included in any oral supplements.

It is not usually sold as a stand alone supplement.

Safety

The Cosmetic Ingredient Review Expert Panel has confirmed that glycyrrhetinic acid is safe for topical administration at concentrations in common use (7).

Licorice itself is included in the FDA GRAS database (Generally Recognized As Safe) at normal levels of consumption (8).

As mentioned previously, excessive oral intake of licorice can cause the syndrome of apparent mineralocorticoid excess which leads to sodium and water retention, hypokalemia and hyperstension. This could be fatal in severe cases.

There is obviously individual variation in susceptibility to the effects of glycyrrhetinic acid and licorice however susceptible individuals can experience adverse effects with daily consumption of 100 mg glycyrrhetinic acid, which corresponds to approximately 50 g liquorice. Using a safety factor of 10 it has been recommended that a maximum safe daily consumption of glycyrrhetinic acid is 10mg or approximately 5g of licorice (9).

Effects on testosterone: Of more interest to the sportsman is the effect of oral intake of glycyrrhetinic acid on testosterone production. Oral intake is associated with decreases in testosterone production both in healthy males and females of up to 44% when consumed in quantities up to 7g. This is due to its ability to inhibit the enzyme 17β-hydroxysteroid dehydrogenase which catalyzes the conversion of androstenedione to testosterone. For obvious reasons I therefore recommend that sportspeople completely avoid consumption of licorice or glycyrrhetinic acid (10) (11) (12).

The topical application of glycyrrhetinic acid is extremely unlikely to reduce testosterone levels. The enzyme 17β-hydroxysteroid dehydrogenase is not present in fat tissue (6).

Interactions

Due to its effect on blood pressure and potassium, glycyrrhetinic acid has the potential to interfere with a variety of medications including blood pressure medications, heart medications such as digoxin and diuretics such as furosemide with potentially serious consequences. In addition it has been seen to reduce the effect of warfarin in animal studies (13). It is advisable that anyone on any kind of medication should not take oral glycyrrhetinic acid without first consulting their doctor.

References

1. Seckl JR, Walker BR. Minireview: 11beta-hydroxysteroid dehydrogenase type 1- a tissue-specific amplifier of glucocorticoid action. Endocrinology. 2001;142(4):1371-6
2. Katz JR, Mohamed-Ali V, Wood PJ, Yudkin JS, Coppack SW. An in vivo study of the cortisol-cortisone shuttle in subcutaneous abdominal adipose tissue. Clin Endocrinol (Oxf). 1999;50(1):63-8

3. Fotsch C, Askew BC, Chen JJ. 11β-Hydroxysteroid dehydrogenase-1 as a therapeutic target for metabolic diseases. Expert Opinion on Therapeutic Patents. 2005;15(3):289-303 [online] at http://informahealthcare.com/doi/abs/10.1517/1354377 6.15.3.289

4. Walker BR, Connacher AA, Lindsay RM, Webb DJ, Edwards CR. Carbenoxolone increases hepatic insulin sensitivity in man: a novel role for 11-oxosteroid reductase in enhancing glucocorticoid receptor activation. J Clin Endocrinol Metab. 1995;80(11):3155-9

5. Armanini D, De Palo CB, Mattarello MJ, Spinella P, Zaccaria M. *et al.* Effect of licorice on the reduction of body fat mass in healthy subjects. J Endocrinol Invest. 2003;26(7):646-50

6. Armanini D, Nacamulli D, Francini-Pesenti F, Battagin G, Ragazzi E, Fiore C. Glycyrrhetinic acid, the active principle of licorice, can reduce the thickness of subcutaneous thigh fat through topical application. Steroids. 2005;70(8):538-42. Epub 2005 Apr 12

7. Cosmetic Ingredient Review Expert Panel. Final report on the safety assessment of Glycyrrhetinic Acid, Potassium Glycyrrhetinate, Disodium Succinoyl Glycyrrhetinate, Glyceryl Glycyrrhetinate, Glycyrrhetinyl Stearate, Stearyl Glycyrrhetinate, Glycyrrhizic Acid, Ammonium Glycyrrhizate, Dipotassium Glycyrrhizate, Disodium Glycyrrhizate, Trisodium Glycyrrhizate, Methyl Glycyrrhizate, and Potassium Glycyrrhizinate. Int J Toxicol. 2007;26 Suppl 2:79-112

8. U.S. Food and Drug Administration. GRAS Substances (SCOGS) Database. [online] at http://www.fda.gov/Food/FoodIngredientsPackaging/G enerallyRecognizedasSafeGRAS/GRASSubstancesSCOG SDatabase/default.htm

9. Størmer FC, Reistad R, Alexander J. Glycyrrhizic acid in liquorice--evaluation of health hazard. Food Chem Toxicol. 1993;31(4):303-12

10. Armanini D, Bonanni G, Palermo M. Reduction of serum testosterone in men by licorice. N Engl J Med. 1999;341(15):1158

11. Armanini D, Bonanni G, Mattarello MJ, Fiore C, Sartorato P, Palermo M. Licorice consumption and serum testosterone in healthy man. Exp Clin Endocrinol Diabetes. 2003;111(6):341-3

12. Armanini D, Mattarello MJ, Fiore C, Bonanni G, Scaroni C, *et al*. Licorice reduces serum testosterone in healthy women. Steroids. 2004 Oct-Nov;69(11-12):763-6

13. Mu Y, Zhang J, Zhang S, Zhou HH, Toma D, *et al*. Traditional Chinese medicines Wu Wei Zi (Schisandra chinensis Baill) and Gan Cao (Glycyrrhiza uralensis Fisch) activate pregnane X receptor and increase warfarin clearance in rats. J Pharmacol Exp Ther. 2006;316(3):1369-77. Epub 2005 Nov 2

Green Tea

Other names

Camellia sinensis
EGCG
Epigallocatechin gallate
Epigallocatechin-3-gallate
Green tea catechins

Star rating

5

What is it?

Tea is made from the leaves of the plant Camellia sinensis. Green tea differs from other types of tea by the manner in which the leaves are processed. Black tea is prepared from leaves which have been crushed and fermented before being dried and oolong tea is from leaves which are partially fermented. Green tea is prepared from unfermented fresh leaves which results in higher levels of catechins which are the active constituents of tea.

Green tea contains 30% or more of catechins while black tea contains 9%. The major catechins present are epicatechin (EC), epicatechin gallate (ECG), epigallocatechin (EGC) and epigallocatechin gallate (EGCG). The usual proportions present are EC 2%, ECG 3%, EGC 10% and EGCG 15%. Studies have shown that EGCG is the most active of the catechins and is responsible for most of the beneficial effects of green tea although the other components also have a small effect and may act synergistically with EGCG. Sports supplements usually contain extracts of green tea standardized to contain a certain amount of EGCG usually between 30-50%.

In addition to catechins tea also contains various other compounds which may contribute to its beneficial effects such as flavonols, theobromine, theophylline, and phenolic acids. Tea also contains approximately 3-6% caffeine (1).

Claimed benefits

Fat loss.

Mode of Action

Green tea is believed to aid weight loss by several different mechanisms. These are reduced fat cell proliferation and growth (2) (3), reduction in absorption of dietary fat via inhibition of gastric and pancreatic lipases (the enzymes which digest fats) (4) possibly reducing food intake by increasing levels of the hormone cholecystokinin which reduces appetite (5) and increasing thermogenesis and fat oxidation (1) (6). Of these by far the most important is increased thermogenesis and fat oxidation. (Thermogenesis is the production of heat by burning fat stores in the body.)

Thermogenesis is under the control of the sympathetic nervous system which controls the secretion of nor-epinephrine (nor-adrenaline) which increases thermogenesis and fat oxidation. In the body nor-epinephrine is broken down by the enzyme catechol-O-methyltransferase (COMT). EGCG in green tea inhibits the action of COMT hence increasing the levels of nor-epinephrine and thermogenesis (1).

Caffeine in green tea or consumed from other sources acts synergistically with EGCG to increase its effect.

Effectiveness

Epidemiological studies (studies of human populations) have shown that regular tea drinkers over a period of more than 10 years have up to 20% less body fat than non tea drinkers (7).

Two recent systematic reviews in 2009 (8) and 2010 (9) analysed all the best studies on green tea supplements and weight loss performed to date. They both concluded that green tea supplements are effective for weight loss and maintaining weight loss, although the 2010 review found that it is only effective if taken together with caffeine. However the amount of weight lost is small.

By way of comparison the 2010 review points out that pharmacological weight loss drugs are expected to produce a weight loss of at least 2kg in 4 weeks to be considered effective. The average weight loss produced by green tea is 1kg over 12 weeks.

Shixian *et al.* (1) calculated that the increase in thermogenesis produced by a green tea supplement was equivalent to burning an extra 75-100kJ of energy per day which over a year would be equivalent to a weight loss of 8lbs or 3.6kg.

Although these numbers are small the weight control effect of green tea does appear to be real and when combined with other weight control ingredients as it usually is in weight loss supplements it is an effective additional tool for weight control.

Commonly used dosages

Green tea is often included as part of a proprietary formulation in commercial sport supplement preparations with the exact quantity of the substance not listed in the ingredients.

It is available as a stand alone supplement usually in capsules of 300-500mg standardized for between 30-50% EGCG.
The average amount of green tea used in most of the weight loss trials was equivalent to a total catechin amount of 400-600mg/day (i.e total amount of EC, ECG, EGC and EGCG).

Peak blood levels of EGCG are reached 1-3 hours after ingestion and the terminal half life is between 2 and 5 hours (10).

Safety

Green tea extracts do not cause increases in heart rate or blood pressure unlike many other weight loss agents (1).

There have been isolated reports of green tea supplements causing liver damage and liver failure. The US Pharmacopeia Dietary Supplement Information Expert Committee systematically reviewed the safety information for green tea products and out of 216 reports of liver damage concluded that 7 were probably caused by use of a green tea supplement.

The toxicological information indicates that consumption of concentrated extracts on an empty stomach is more likely to cause liver problems than consumption with food. They concluded that the health risk from green tea supplements is low provided they are consumed with food and supplement labels should include a recommendation to this effect (11).

Interactions

Green tea catechins have been reported to have anti-platelet activity which could slow blood clotting. There is a theoretical risk that green tea and green tea supplements could increase the risk of bleeding if taken with antiplatelet or anticoagulant drugs such as aspirin, clopidogrel or warfarin and people taking these kinds of medicines should avoid green tea (12).

Green tea is often promoted for its anti-cancer effects however EGCG and other polyphenols in green tea can block the action of the anti-cancer drug bortezomib used in the treatment of multiple myeloma. Patients on this drug or other drugs in this class called boronic acid-based proteasome inhibitors should not take green tea or green tea supplements (13).

The caffeine content of green tea has a variety of interactions with other drugs and medicines, however since the amount of caffeine in green tea is quite low this is unlikely to be significant. An 8 ounce cup of green tea contains 9-50mg of caffeine compared to 72-130mg in an 8 ounce cup of coffee (14). However care should be taken if large amounts of supplements are taken or if green tea is taken as part of a combination weight loss supplement which usually also contain caffeine. See the entry on caffeine in this book for detailed advice on drug interactions of caffeine.

References

1. Shixian Q, VanCrey B, Shi J, Kakuda Y, Jiang Y. Green tea extract thermogenesis-induced weight loss by epigallocatechin gallate inhibition of catechol-O-methyltransferase. J Med Food. 2006;9(4):451-8
2. Wolfram S, Wang Y, Thielecke F. Anti-obesity effects of green tea: from bedside to bench. Mol Nutr Food Res. 2006;50(2):176-87
3. Mori M, Hasegawa N. Superoxide dismutase activity enhanced by green tea inhibits lipid accumulation in 3T3-L1 cells. Phytother Res. 2003;17(5):566-7
4. Chantre P, Lairon D. Recent findings of green tea extract AR25 (Exolise) and its activity for the treatment of obesity. Phytomedicine. 2002;9(1):3-8
5. Liao S. The medicinal action of androgens and green tea epigallocatechin gallate. Hong Kong Med J. 2001;7(4):369-74
6. Dulloo AG, Duret C, Rohrer D, Girardier L, Mensi N *et al.* Efficacy of a green tea extract rich in catechin polyphenols and caffeine in increasing 24-h energy

expenditure and fat oxidation in humans. Am J Clin Nutr. 1999;70(6):1040-5

7. Wu CH, Lu FH, Chang CS, Chang TC, Wang RH, Chang CJ. Relationship among habitual tea consumption, percent body fat, and body fat distribution. Obes Res. 2003;11(9):1088-95

8. Hursel R, Viechtbauer W, Westerterp-Plantenga MS. The effects of green tea on weight loss and weight maintenance: a meta-analysis. Int J Obes (Lond). 2009;33(9):956-61. Epub 2009 Jul 14

9. Phung OJ, Baker WL, Matthews LJ, Lanosa M, Thorne A, Coleman CI. Effect of green tea catechins with or without caffeine on anthropometric measures: a systematic review and meta-analysis. Am J Clin Nutr. 2010;91(1):73-81. Epub 2009 Nov 11

10. Nagle DG, Ferreira D, Zhou YD. Epigallocatechin-3-gallate (EGCG): chemical and biomedical perspectives. Phytochemistry. 2006;67(17):1849-55. Epub 2006 Jul 31

11. Sarma DN, Barrett ML, Chavez ML, Gardiner P, Ko R *et al*. Safety of green tea extracts : a systematic review by the US Pharmacopeia. Drug Saf. 2008;31(6):469-84

12. Son DJ, Cho MR, Jin YR, Kim SY, Park YH *et al*. Antiplatelet effect of green tea catechins: a possible mechanism through arachidonic acid pathway. Prostaglandins Leukot Essent Fatty Acids. 2004;71(1):25-31

13. Golden EB, Lam PY, Kardosh A, Gaffney KJ, Cadenas E *et al*. Green tea polyphenols block the anticancer effects of bortezomib and other boronic acid-based proteasome inhibitors. Blood. 2009;113(23):5927-37. Epub 2009 Feb 3

14. Oregon State University. Linus Pauling Institute. Micronutrient Information Center – Tea. [online] at http://lpi.oregonstate.edu/infocenter/phytochemicals/tea/#components

Guanidinopropionic Acid

Other names

β-Guanadinopropionate
β-Guanidinopropionic acid
3-(diaminomethylideneamino)propanoic acid
3-carbamimidamidopropanoic acid
3-Guanidinopropanoate
3-Guanidinopropionic acid
3-Guanidino-propionic acid

Star rating

2

What is it?

A creatine analogue.

Claimed benefits

Fat loss.
Improved body composition, i.e. more lean muscle mass and less fat mass.
Improved creatine uptake.

Mode of Action

Guanidinoproprionic acid improves insulin sensitivity by increasing the ability of the insulin-responsive glucose transporter GLUT-4 to transport glucose into muscle cells. It probably does this by increasing the numbers of GLUT-4 transporter molecules on the cell surface (1).

Effectiveness

Guanidinoproprionic acid has been shown to increase glucose transport activity by 40% to 50% in *in vivo* studies with rats.

It has also been shown to effectively improve insulin sensitivity and reduce fat tissue in non-insulin dependent diabetic animals such as mice and rhesus monkeys (2) (3) (4). However it has no effect in healthy normoglycemic animals (4).

Contrary to popular claims on the internet, guanidinoproprionic acid does NOT increase creatine uptake but rather it inhibits it. This is because guanidinoproprionic acid competes with creatine for entry to the creatine transport site (5).

Commonly used dosages

Guanidinoproprionic acid is usually included as part of a proprietary formulation in commercial sport supplement preparations with the exact quantity of the substance not listed in the ingredients.

It is not usually sold as a stand alone supplement.

Safety

The short and long term safety effects of depletion of muscle creatine are unknown. The depletion of muscle creatine by guanidinoproprionic acid has also been observed in the heart in tests on rats where it has been observed to impair cardiac function and possibly cause cardiac damage due to a disruption of the creatine kinase energy circuit (6) (7).

In other studies on rats, guanidinoproprionic acid has also been shown to downregulate AMP-D activity by up to 80% in fast twitch muscle fibres (7). AMP-D (Adenosine Monophosphate Deaminase) is an essential enzyme for the production of energy in muscle cells. Deficiency of AMP-D is a known cause of exercise-induced myopathy and probably the most common cause of metabolic myopathy in man (8).

Due to its potentially adverse effects and lack of safety data in humans the use of supplements containing guanidinoproprionic acid cannot be recommended.

Interactions

None known.

References

1. Ren JM, Semenkovich CF, Holloszy JO. Adaptation of muscle to creatine depletion: effect on GLUT-4 glucose transporter expression. Am J Physiol. 1993;264(1 Pt 1):C146-50
2. Vaillancourt VA, Larsen SD, Tanis SP, Burr JE, Connell MA, *et al.* Synthesis and biological activity of aminoguanidine and diaminoguanidine analogues of the antidiabetic/antiobesity agent 3-guanidinopropionic acid. J Med Chem. 2001;44(8):1231-48
3. Larsen SD, Connell MA, Cudahy MM, Evans BR, May PD, *et al.* Synthesis and biological activity of analogues of the antidiabetic/antiobesity agent 3-guanidinopropionic acid: discovery of a novel aminoguanidinoacetic acid antidiabetic agent. J Med Chem. 2001;44(8):1217-30
4. Meglasson MD, Wilson JM, Yu JH, Robinson DD, Wyse BM, de Souza CJ. Antihyperglycemic action of guanidinoalkanoic acids: 3-guanidinopropionic acid ameliorates hyperglycemia in diabetic KKAy and

C57BL6Job/ob mice and increases glucose disappearance in rhesus monkeys. J Pharmacol Exp Ther. 1993 Sep;266(3):1454-62
5. Fitch CD, Shields RP, Payne WF, Dacus JM. Creatine metabolism in skeletal muscle. 3. Specificity of the creatine entry process. J Biol Chem. 1968;243(8):2024-7
6. Clark JF, Khuchua Z, Kuznetsov AV, Vassil'eva E, Boehm E, *et al.* Actions of the creatine analogue beta-guanidinopropionic acid on rat heart mitochondria. Biochem J. 1994 May 15;300 (Pt 1):211-6
7. Tullson PC, Rundell KW, Sabina RL, Terjung RL. Creatine analogue beta-guanidinopropionic acid alters skeletal muscle AMP deaminase activity. Am J Physiol. 1996;270(1 Pt 1):C76-85
8. Sabina RL, Fishbein WN, Pezeshkpour G, Clarke PR, Holmes EW. Molecular analysis of the myoadenylate deaminase deficiencies. Neurology. 1992;42(1):170-9

Guarana

Other names

Brazilian cocoa
Guarana bread
Paullinia cupana
Zoom

Star rating

3

What is it?

A rainforest vine in the family Sapindaceae (scientific name

Paullinia cupana) common in the Amazon, particularly Brazil. The seeds are about the size of coffee beans but contain between 2% to 7.5% caffeine which is up to four times as much as coffee beans (1). They also contain theobromine, theophylline and up to 16% tannins (2).

The caffeine found in guarana is sometimes referred to as guaranine. There has been some debate as to whether guaranine is a structurally different form of caffeine, however it is now generally accepted that guaranine should be considered an impure form of caffeine and is probably caffeine bound to another tannin or phenol constituent of guarana (3).

Claimed benefits

Fat loss.
Improved endurance.

Mode of Action

Most of the effects of guarana come from its caffeine content (2) (see separate entry for caffeine).

However there is some evidence that guarana may have a small effect independent of caffeine to increase physical capacity (4) and to improve cognition (5) (6), although the mechanism or constituents responsible for this are currently unknown.

Effectiveness

See also separate entry for caffeine.

There are a few small human studies which show guarana to be effective for weight loss when combined with other herbal ingredients such as Ma Huang, Yerbe Maté and Damiana (7) (8).

Unfortuantely there are very few studies which evaluate guarana alone. In tests on mice guarana was effective at preventing exercise induced hypoglycemia (9) and was also effective at increasing swimming times (4). In another study using guarana fed rats, guarana was effective at reducing body fat, however the study concluded that this effect was due to the caffeine content of guarana since rats fed decaffeinated guarana did not experience similar results (2).

Commonly used dosages

There is a wide variation in dosages of guarana included in sport supplements, from as little as 12mg up to 700mg. Guarana is not usually sold as a stand alone supplement except in the form of energy drinks, of which there are now many guarana based drinks on the market.

Safety

See entry for caffeine.

Interactions

See entry for caffeine.

References

1. Smith N, Atroch AL. Guarana's Journey from Regional Tonic to Aphrodisiac and Global Energy Drink. Evid Based Complement Alternat Med. 2007 Dec 5. [Epub ahead of print]
2. Lima WP, Carnevali LC Jr, Eder R, Costa Rosa LF, Bacchi EM, Seelaender MC. Lipid metabolism in trained rats:

effect of guarana (Paullinia cupana Mart.) supplementation. Clin Nutr. 2005;24(6):1019-28. Epub 2005 Sep 22

3. MDidea. Guarana and Gurana Extract:Phytochemicals,Botanical Info and History. [online] at http://www.mdidea.com/products/proper/proper04802.html

4. Espinola EB, Dias RF, Mattei R, Carlini EA. Pharmacological activity of Guarana (Paullinia cupana Mart.) in laboratory animals. J Ethnopharmacol. 1997;55(3):223-9

5. Haskell CF, Kennedy DO, Wesnes KA, Milne AL, Scholey AB A double-blind, placebo-controlled, multi-dose evaluation of the acute behavioural effects of guaraná in humans. J Psychopharmacol. 2007;21(1):65-70. Epub 2006 Mar 13

6. .Kennedy DO, Haskell CF, Wesnes KA, Scholey AB. Improved cognitive performance in human volunteers following administration of guarana (Paullinia cupana) extract: comparison and interaction with Panax ginseng. Pharmacol Biochem Behav. 2004;79(3):401-11

7. Andersen T, Fogh J. Weight loss and delayed gastric emptying following a South American herbal preparation in overweight patients. J Hum Nutr Diet. 2001;14(3):243-50

8. Boozer CN, Nasser JA, Heymsfield SB, Wang V, Chen G, Solomon JL. An herbal supplement containing Ma Huang-Guarana for weight loss: a randomized, double-blind trial. Int J Obes Relat Metab Disord. 2001;25(3):316-24

9. Miura T, Tatara M, Nakamura K, Suzuki I. Effect of guarana on exercise in normal and epinephrine-induced glycogenolytic mice. Biol Pharm Bull. 1998;21(6):646-8

Guggulsterones E & Z

Other names

Balsamodendrum mukul
Balsamodendrum wightii
Commiphora Mukul
Commiphora wightii
Guggul
Guggul Gum
Guggul Lipids
Indian Bdellium
Pregna-4,17(20)-diene-3,16-dione

Star rating

3

What is it?

The gum resin of the Ayurvedic medicinal plant Commiphora mukul contains a plant sterol called guggulsterone. Guggulsterone exists in two naturally occurring isomeric forms, the E-isomer and the Z-isomer, both of which are biologically active (1).

Claimed benefits

Weight loss.

Mode of Action

Guggulsterones have been shown to increase thyroid activity in animal models (2), (3) and counteract the thyroid-suppressant activity of a known thyroid inhibitor (4). It appears that the thyroid is stimulated to produce more of the hormone T3 (tri-iodothyronine) and the peripheral conversion of T4 (thyroxine) to T3 is also facilitated (5).

Effectiveness

Few human studies have been conducted to assess the effectiveness of guggulsterones as a weight loss aid but those which have show promise.

In one study involving 20 subjects, 6 received a combination of guggulsterones, hydroxycitric acid (*garcinia cambogia*) and L-tyrosine while the remaining subjects were divided into control and placebo groups. All groups also undertook exercise and dietary restriction. After 6 weeks the guggulsterone group had lost 4.3kg of fat compared to only 1.5kg and 1.4kg in the control and placebo groups respectively. Three of the subjects in the guggulsterone group had their T3 levels measured and two of them had an 8 – 10% increase but the third showed no change (6).

In a larger study of 58 obese subjects half were given guggulsterones and half a placebo. All subjects undertook an exercise regime and dietary restriction. The mean difference in weight loss between the guggulsterone group and the placebo group was 0.32 kg on day 15 and 0.58 kg on day 30, showing the guggulsterone group had lost more fat although the result did not reach statistical significance (7).

Commonly used dosages

1000mg to 2000mg standardized to contain 75 – 150mg of guggulsterones taken 2 or 3 times daily have been commonly used dosages in trials.

Safety

Should be avoided by pregnant women. May stimulate menstrual flow and uterine contractions which could cause miscarriage (8).

Interactions

Guggulsterones may inhibit platelet aggregation and so taking it with antiplatelet or anticoagulant drugs such as aspirin, diclofenac etc. might increase the risk of bruising and bleeding (9).

Guggulsterones may have estrogen-alpha receptor agonist activity and may increase the effects of medications having estrogenic activity including contraceptives and hormone replacement therapy or reduce the effects of estrogen antagonising drugs such as Tamoxifen (Nolvadex) (10).

References

1. The Merck Index 14th Ed. New Jersey, Merck & Co. Inc. 2006.
2. Tripathi YB, Malhotra OP, Tripathi SN. Thyroid stimulating action of Z-guggulsterone obtained from Commiphora mukul. Planta Med. 1984 Feb;50(1):78-80.
3. Panda S, Kar A. Guggulu (Commiphora mukul) potentially ameliorates hypothyroidism in female mice. Phytother Res. 2005 Jan;19(1):78-80.
4. Tripathi YB, Tripathi P, Malhotra OP, Tripathi SN. Thyroid stimulatory action of (Z)-guggulsterone: mechanism of action. Planta Med 1988;54:271-7.
5. Panda S, Kar A. Gugulu (Commiphora mukul) induces triiodothyronine production: possible involvement of lipid peroxidation. Life Sci 1999;65:PL137-41.

6. Antonio J, Colker CM, Torina GC, et al. Effects of a standardized guggulsterone phosphate supplement on body composition in overweight adults: a pilot study. Curr Ther Res 1999;60:220-7.

7. Bhatt AD, Dalal DG, Shah SJ, Joshi BA, Gajjar MN, Vaidya RA, Vaidya AB, Antarkar DS. Conceptual and methodologic challenges of assessing the short-term efficacy of Guggulu in obesity: data emergent from a naturalistic clinical trial. J Postgrad Med 1995 Jan-Mar;41(1):5-7

8. Drug Digest [online] at http://www.drugdigest.org/DD/DVH/HerbsCareful/0,3 924,552123%7CGuggal%2BResin,00.html

9. Mester L, Mester M, Nityanand S. Inhibition of platelet aggregation by "guggulu" steroids. Planta Med 1979;37:367-9.

10. Brobst DE, Ding X, Creech KL, et al. Guggulsterone activates multiple nuclear receptors and induces CYP3A gene expression through the pregnane X receptor. J Pharmacol Exp Ther 2004;310:528-35

Gynostemma

Other names

Amachazuru
Dungkulcha
Fairy herb
Gynostemma pedatum
Gynostemma pentaphyllum
Jiao Chu Lan
Jiao Gu Lan
Jioagulan
Miracle grass
Penta tea
Southern ginseng
Vitis pentaphylla
Xiancao

Star rating

2

What is it?

A herbaceous perennial vine of the Cucurbitaceae family native to China, Japan and Korea. It is used in Chinese medicine, the earliest known mention of the herb being in a book of botany called *Zhi Wu Ming Shi Tu Kao Chang Bian* written in 1848 by Wu Qijun.

Claimed benefits

Increases strength and endurance.
Is an "adaptogen" i.e. it increases the body's resistance to stress and fatigue by modulating endocrine hormones and the immune system.

Mode of Action

The mode of action is unclear. A large number of compounds called dammarane triterpene saponins (referred to as gypenosides when extracted from Gynostemma) have been isolated from Gynostemma many of which are identical to the supposedly adaptogenic saponins found in Ginseng. For example, gypenoside 3 is structurally identical to ginsenoside Rb1, likewise gypenoside 4 is identical to ginsenoside Rb3, gypenoside 8 is identical to ginsenoside Rd, and gypenoside 12 is equivalent to ginsenoside F2 (1).

Effectiveness

There are various cell and animal studies indicating that Gynostemma may have a number of beneficial effects on health. For example it has been shown to have anti-oxidant activity and protect the cardiovascular system against atherosclerosis and arrhythmias (2) (3), it can reduce bronchoconstriction in the lungs (4), it can reduce oxidative stress against various types of cells, including white blood cells, endothelial cells and liver cells (5), it reduces cholesterol and triglycerides (6), it releases nitric oxide and promotes vasodilation (7) and it can improve immune function (8).

Taken together these animal studies carried out so far do therefore show some evidence to support the claim that Gynostemma functions as an adaptogen, however it is still uncertain to what extent this would improve endurance, strength or sporting performance.

I have only been able to identify one Chinese study which specifically tested for the effect of Gynostemma on endurance. This study, which was again an animal study using mice, showed that Gynostemma increased exercise endurance and improved recovery from exercise (9) (details taken from study abstract only as the full study is in Chinese).

There do not appear to be any human studies evaluating Gynostemma as an adaptogen although Chinese human studies have confirmed the cholesterol lowering and immune system enhancing effects (1).

Commonly used dosages

Gynostemma is usually included as part of a proprietary formulation in commercial sport supplement preparations with the exact quantity of the substance not listed in the ingredients.

It is possible to buy Gynostemma as a stand alone supplement usually in tablets or capsules from 250mg to 500mg. Sometimes manufacturers state that the extract is standardized to contain a standard amount of gypenosides, often from 10% to 30%.

In the above mentioned human trials which showed Gynostemma to be useful in the treatment of hypercholesterolemia, the subjects are reported to have received 10mg three times a day.

Safety

Gypenoside 3 a constituent of Gynostemma is structurally identical to ginsenoside Rb1 which has been shown to cause birth defects in rat embryos. Gynostemma should therefore be avoided in pregnancy (10).

Interactions

Gynostemma has been shown to inhibit platelet aggregation in human blood samples which could increase bruising and bleeding times (11). It could theoretically increase the effect of anti-platelet and anti-clotting drugs such such as aspirin and warfarin. It should therefore be avoided by anyone taking these classes of drugs.

References

1. Drugs.com. Jiaogulan. [online] at http://www.drugs.com/npp/jiaogulan.html
2. Li L, Lau BHS. Protection of vascular endothelial cells from hydrogen peroxide-induced oxidant injury by gypenosides, saponins of Gynostemma pentaphyllum. Phytother Res 1993;7(4):299-304
3. Circosta C, De Pasquale R, Occhiuto F. Cardiovascular effects of the aqueous extract of Gynostemma pentaphyllum Makino. Phytomedicine. 2005;12(9):638-43
4. Circosta C, De Pasquale R, Palumbo DR, Occhiuto F. Bronchodilatory effects of the aqueous extract of Gynostemma pentaphyllum and gypenosides III and VIII in anaesthetized guinea-pigs. J Pharm Pharmacol. 2005;57(8):1053-8
5. Li L, Jiao L, Lau BH. Protective effect of gypenosides against oxidative stress in phagocytes, vascular endothelial cells and liver microsomes. Cancer Biother. 1993;8(3):263-72
6. Megalli S, Aktan F, Davies NM, Roufogalis BD. Phytopreventative anti-hyperlipidemic effects of gynostemma pentaphyllum in rats. J Pharm Pharm Sci. 2005;8(3):507-15
7. Tanner MA, Bu X, Steimle JA, Myers PR. The direct release of nitric oxide by gypenosides derived from the

herb Gynostemma pentaphyllum. Nitric Oxide. 1999;3(5):359-65

8. Hau DM, Feng Y, Chen WC, Lin IH, Chen KT, *et al.* Effects of gypenosides on cellular immunity of gamma-ray-irradiated mice. Chin Med J (Engl). 1996;109(2):143-6
9. FU Yi. The Experimental Study for Gynostemma pentaphyllum With Sport Endurance. Journal of Chengdu Physical Education Institute. 2000-02
10. Chan LY, Chiu PY, Lau TK. An in-vitro study of ginsenoside Rb1-induced teratogenicity using a whole rat embryo culture model. Hum Reprod. 2003;18(10):2166-8
11. Tan H, Liu ZL, Liu MJ. [Antithrombotic effect of Gynostemma pentaphyllum] [Article in Chinese] Zhongguo Zhong Xi Yi Jie He Za Zhi. 1993;13(5):278-80, 261

HCA

Other names

(1S,2S)-1,2-dihydroxypropane-1,2,3-tricarboxylic acid
(2S,3S)-3-Carboxy-2,3-dihydroxy-pentanedioic acid
Brindall berry
Brindleberry
Garcinia acid
Garcinia Cambogia
Garcinia gummi-guta
Garcinia Quaesita
Hydroxycitrate
Hydroxycitric acid
Malabar tamarind

Star rating

2

What is it?

The active compound derived from the rind of the tropical plant Garcinia Cambogia but also found in Garcinia Indica and Hibiscus subdariffa. The rind of Garcinia Camobogia contains 10-30% HCA (1).

Claimed benefits

Weight loss.

Mode of Action

HCA inhibits the enzyme adenosine triphosphate–citrate (pro-3S)-lyase which is involved in converting excess blood glucose into fat for storage. HCA therefore promotes fat burning for energy.

Research on animals suggests that HCA may also suppress appetite (1) (2).

Effectiveness

A few early studies in the 1990's appeared to show promising results for HCA as a weight loss agent. However most of these studies suffered from drawbacks such as administering HCA in combination with other substances, no placebo control, small numbers of subjects participating etc.

All of the larger well designed studies performed since then have shown that HCA is ineffective for weight loss (3) (4) does not increase the rate at which fat is utilized for energy

(5) and does not suppress appetite or increase feelings of satiety (6) (7).

Commonly used dosages

It is important when considering doses to differentiate between amount of HCA and amount of Garcinia Cambogia extract containing HCA. Sport supplements usually state containing HCA in the ingredients in varying amounts from 150mg to1000mg.

Garcinia Cambogia extract is usually stated on the ingredients for diet supplements with amounts from 1000mg to 2000mg being common and is often standardized to contain 50% or 60% HCA.

Most of the studies mentioned above used 1500mg to 3000mg of HCA per day.

Safety

No known safety issues.

Interactions

None known.

References

1. Soni MG, Burdock GA, Preuss HG, Stohs SJ, Ohia SE, Bagchi D. Safety assessment of (-)-hydroxycitric acid and Super CitriMax, a novel calcium/potassium salt. Food Chem Toxicol. 2004;42(9):1513-29
2. Sullivan AC, Triscari J, Hamilton JG, Miller ON. Effect of (-)-hydroxycitrate upon the accumulation of lipid in the rat. II. Appetite. Lipids. 1974;9(2):129-34

3. Heymsfield SB, Allison DB, Vasselli JR, Pietrobelli A, Greenfield D, Nunez C. Garcinia cambogia (hydroxycitric acid) as a potential antiobesity agent: a randomized controlled trial. JAMA. 1998;280(18):1596-600

4. Vasques CA, Rossetto S, Halmenschlager G, Linden R, Heckler E *et al*. Evaluation of the pharmacotherapeutic efficacy of Garcinia cambogia plus Amorphophallus konjac for the treatment of obesity. Phytother Res. 2008;22(9):1135-40

5. Kriketos AD, Thompson HR, Greene H, Hill JO. (-)-Hydroxycitric acid does not affect energy expenditure and substrate oxidation in adult males in a post-absorptive state. Int J Obes Relat Metab Disord. 1999;23(8):867-73

6. Mattes RD, Bormann L. Effects of (-)-hydroxycitric acid on appetitive variables. Physiol Behav. 2000 Oct;71(1-2):87-94

7. Kovacs EM, Westerterp-Plantenga MS, de Vries M, Brouns F, Saris WH. Effects of 2-week ingestion of (-)-hydroxycitrate and (-)-hydroxycitrate combined with medium-chain triglycerides on satiety and food intake. Physiol Behav. 2001;74(4-5):543-9

HMB

Other names

β-Hydroxy β-Methylbutyrate Monohydrate
β-Hydroxy-β-Methylbutyric Acid
Calcium β-Hydroxy β-Methylbutyrate Monohydrate
Hydroxymethylbutyrate

Star rating

4

What is it?

A metabolite of the branched chain amino acid leucine which is formed in the cytosol of cells by the enzyme a-ketoisocaproate dioxygenase. Approximately 5% of leucine is converted into HMB. An average person produces about 0.2-0.4g of HMB per day naturally in the body (1).

HMB is also present naturally in small amounts in certain foods such as grapefruit and catfish (2).

Claimed benefits

Increased muscle mass via both anti-catabolic and anabolic actions.

Fat loss.

Mode of Action

The exact mode of action is not known however various theories have been proposed (1) (2) (3) some or all of which may play a role:

1. Increased muscle fibre protein synthesis via a similar mechanism of action to leucine.
2. Reduced muscle fibre breakdown via down-regulation of a mechanism called the ubiquitin pathway.
3. HMB increases muscle cell cholesterol synthesis which stabilises the muscle cell membrane and is important for muscle cell growth.
4. Recent research in mice shows HMB can increase production of the anabolic hormone IGF-1 in the liver (1).
5. For fat loss it is proposed that HMB increases the rate at which muscle cells use fatty acids for energy.

Effectiveness

There have been many studies on HMB involving both animals and humans. Of the human studies the effects of HMB have been investigated in both trained and untrained athletes in a variety of sports including resistance training. The effects of HMB have also been evaluated in a variety of studies on patients suffering from various muscle wasting disease states.

Fortunately we do not have to analyse all this evidence since there have been four major papers which have already carried out this process, two large reviews (1) (2) and two meta analyses (3) (4).

The results of these four papers can be summarised as follows:

There is a clear but small benefit to untrained weight lifters from HMB supplementation. In these individuals lower body strength gains appear to be greater than upper body strength gains, however there is a clear overall increase in average strength. In trained lifters the benefit is less clear, there appears to be a definite positive effect however it is extremely small. One of the meta analyses (4) calculated an average strength gain of 1.4% per week and a lean mass gain of 0.28% per week (average of trained and untrained lifters).

Possible reasons for discrepancies in the response between trained and untrained lifters may be found in the design of some studies. HMB seems to have optimal effects in catabolic states such as those generated during intense exercise. Trained individuals require a greater training stimulus to elicit muscle damage and some study training protocols do not seem to have been sufficiently demanding to elicit this effect. Furthermore some of the studies may have been of insufficient duration to measure significant benefits in trained individuals compared to untrained individuals who typically have a faster response to initial periods of training.

Finally it should be noted that according to one study the effects of HMB and creatine are additive and produce greater gains in lean body mass and strength than either supplement used alone (5).

Regarding the fat loss effects of HMB a separate systematic review which specifically evaluated the ability of HMB to reduce fat mass from four randomised controlled trials concluded that in all the trials evaluated there was a tendency to increase lean body mass but that more studies were needed to confirm these results (6).

Commonly used dosages

HMB is included in a variety of sport supplements but is usually sold as a stand-alone supplement in capsules containing 1000mg HMB.

Virtually all studies on HMB used a dose of 3g per day. Studies using higher doses (up to 6g/day) have found no additional benefit over the 3g dose.

HMB has a half life of 2.5 hours and after consumption reaches baseline levels again after 9 hours which suggests the optimum pattern of consumption is 1g taken 3 times daily. It does not seem to make any difference whether HMB is consumed pre or post exercise (2).

Safety

No known safety issues.

Interactions

None known.

References

1. Zanchi NE, Gerlinger-Romero F, Guimarães-Ferreira L, de Siqueira Filho MA, Felitti V *et al.* HMB supplementation: clinical and athletic performance-related effects and mechanisms of action. Amino Acids. 2010 Jul 6. [Epub ahead of print]
2. Wilson GJ, Wilson JM, Manninen AH. Effects of beta-hydroxy-beta-methylbutyrate (HMB) on exercise performance and body composition across varying levels of age, sex, and training experience: A review. Nutr Metab (Lond). 2008;5:1
3. Rowlands DS, Thomson JS. Effects of beta-hydroxy-beta-methylbutyrate supplementation during resistance training on strength, body composition, and muscle damage in trained and untrained young men: a meta-analysis. J Strength Cond Res. 2009;23(3):836-46

4. Nissen SL, Sharp RL. Effect of dietary supplements on lean mass and strength gains with resistance exercise: a meta-analysis. J Appl Physiol. 2003;94(2):651-9. Epub 2002 Oct 25

5. Jówko E, Ostaszewski P, Jank M, Sacharuk J, Zieniewicz A *et al*. Creatine and beta-hydroxy-beta-methylbutyrate (HMB) additively increase lean body mass and muscle strength during a weight-training program. Nutrition. 2001;17(7-8):558-66

6. Pittler MH, Ernst E. Dietary supplements for body-weight reduction: a systematic review. Am J Clin Nutr. 2004;79(4):529-36

Hoodia

Other names

Bushman's hat
Hoodia Gordonii
Hoodia Pilifera

Star rating

2

What is it?

Hoodia is a genus of plants containing 13 species belonging to the family Apocynaceae. They are cactus like succulents which grow in South Africa and Namibia. One species, Hoodia Gordonii, is used as a traditional medicine by the indigenous San people of South Africa as an appetite suppressant, thirst quencher and remedy for various minor ailments.

Claimed benefits

Weight loss.

Mode of Action

Two species, Hoodia Gordonii and Hoodia Pilifera, have been found to contain an appetite suppressing compound a pregnane glycoside having the structure 3β-[β-d-thevetopyranosyl-(1→4)-β-d- cymaropyranosyl-(1→4)-β-d-cymaropyranosyloxy]-12β-tigloyloxy-14β-hydroxypregn-5-en-20-one. This compound has been named P57 (1).

In a US patent filed by the South African Council for Scientific and Industrial Research (CSIR) who discovered P57 they state that they believe P57 acts as an agonist of the melanocortin 4 receptor which regulates neuropeptide Y and also increases cholecystokinin. Cholecystokinin delays gastric emptying and neuropeptide Y is a regulator of feeding behaviour (2).

Effectiveness

Hoodia has been shown to suppress appetite in rats (1) in research conducted by CSIR.

In 1997 CSIR began collaborating with a British company called Phytopharm plc for the worldwide development of P57. The following year Phytopharm licensed the pharmaceutical giant Pfizer to continue developing the compound, however after five years Pfizer discontinued development in 2003 for reasons which are unclear (3).

In 2004 P57 was then licensed to British food and home products giant Unilever plc for use in its Slimfast weight management range. However once again in 2008 Unilever discontinued development of P57 saying it did not meet their safety and efficacy standards (4).

Commonly used dosages

Hoodia can be found in sport supplements in doses ranging from 100mg to 500mg. It can also be purchased as a stand alone product in similar doses.

There is no research available indicating effective doses in humans.

Safety

No known safety issues but see the comments made by Unilever (above) who discontinued development of Hoodia in 2008.

Interactions

None known.

References

1. Vleggaar R, Senabe JV, Gunning PJ. An appetite suppressant from Hoodia species. Phytochemistry 2007;68(20): 2545-2553
2. United States Patent & Trademark Office, Patent Full Text & Image Database, United States Patent 6,376,657 [online] at http://patft.uspto.gov/netacgi/nph-Parser?Sect1=PTO1&Sect2=HITOFF&d=PALL&p=1&u=%2Fnetahtml%2FPTO%2Fsrchnum.htm&r=1&f=G&l=50&s1=6376657.PN.&OS=PN/6376657&RS=PN/6376657
3. Press Release by Phytopharm plc. Pfizer returns rights of P57. [online] at http://www.phytopharm.com/pfizer-returns-rights-of-p5/

4. Food and Drink Europe.com Unilever drops hoodia. [online] at http://www.foodanddrinkeurope.com/Products-Marketing/Unilever-drops-hoodia

Hordenine

Other names

4-[2-(Dimethylamino)ethyl]phenol
Anhalin
Anhaline
Cactine
Eremursine
Hordenin
N,N-Dimethyltyramine
p-(2-Dimethylaminoethyl)phenol
Peyocactine
p-hydroxy-N,N-dimethylphenethylamine

Star rating

2

What is it?

A dimethyl tyramine produced in nature by several varieties of plants in the Cactacea family. The main source of hordenine in the human diet is beer brewed from barley.

Claimed benefits

Weight loss.

Mode of Action

Hordenine is a central nervous system stimulant (1). Some sources say this is an indirect effect due to its ability to stimulate the release of norepinephrine (noradrenaline) (2) while other sources say hordenine has a direct effect by directly stimulating the norepinephrine receptor i.e. it is an adrenergic receptor agonist (3).

Norepinephrine is a lipolytic hormone, meaning it helps to release fats from adipose tissue to be burned for energy.

Effectiveness

Hordenine has only been tested in animals (2) (4) and its effects have been seen to be short lived and only evident after intravenous administration while oral supplementation had no effect.

Commonly used dosages

Hordenine is usually included as part of a proprietary formulation in commercial sport supplement preparations with the exact quantity of the substance not listed in the ingredients.

It is not usually available as a stand alone supplement.

Safety

No known safety issues.

Interactions

None known.

References

1. Schweitzer A, Wright S. Action of hordenine compounds on the central nervous system. J Physiol. 1938;92(4):422-38
2. Hapke HJ, Strathmann W. [Pharmacological effects of hordenine] Dtsch Tierarztl Wochenschr. 1995;102(6):228-32
3. National Center for Biotechnology Information, PubChem Compound, Hordenine. [online] at http://pubchem.ncbi.nlm.nih.gov/summary/summary.c gi?cid=68313&loc=ec_rcs
4. Frank M, Weckman TJ, Wood T, Woods WE, Tai CL *et al*. Hordenine: pharmacology, pharmacokinetics and behavioural effects in the horse. Equine Vet J. 1990;22(6):437-41

Humulus Lupulus

Other names

Common hop
Hops
Lupulin
Lupulinum
Lupulus

Star rating

1

What is it?

A herbaceous plant commonly called hops, the flower cones

of which are used in the manufacture of beer.

Claimed benefits

Appetite enhancer.
Stimulant.

Mode of Action

Soft resins derived from hops contain the bitter principles α acid humulone and β acid lupulone which are claimed to be responsible for the appetite stimulating effect.

A powder obtained from sifting dried hops and known in herbal medicine as lupulinum is claimed to be responsible for the stimulatory effect.

Effectiveness

Both of these claimed activities of hops derive from traditional herbal medicine and there is no modern scientific evidence supporting them. The claimed appetite stimulating activity is mentioned in herbal works such as King's American Dispensatory 1898 (1) and The British Pharmaceutical Codex 1907 (2).

A phrase which often appears in sport supplement promotional material promoting the stimulatory effects of hops appears to derive from a sentence in King's American Dispensatory regarding lupulinum which states "It produces at first a stimulant influence, succeded by a very agreeable, calming sensation..." (3)

It should be pointed out however that whatever stimulatory properties hops possess they are better known in herbal medicine for their sedative properties. There is evidence from both animal and human studies that they do indeed possess sedative effects so hops are probably best avoided by those seeking a stimulant (4) (5) (6).

Of further interest to the athlete or sports person is the fact that hops contain one of the most potent known plant phytoestrogens which has been identified as the prenylflavanone, 8-prenylnaringenin (8-PN) (7).

Compared to human estrogen (β-estradiol) and another well known phytoestrogen genistein, 8-PN is between 5-23 x less potent than β-estradiol but 7-50 x more potent than genistein (depending on how you measure the estrogenic activity).

Given this it is not surprising to find that herbal preparations containing hops are frequently marketed for the relief of post menopausal symptoms in women.

Beer also contains small quantities of 8-PN however the estrogenic activity of beer is only equivalent to a few μg of β-estradiol.

For the above reasons I recommend that sports people avoid any supplements containing hops and the excessive consumption of beer.

Commonly used dosages

Sport supplements usually contain approximately 1000mg humulus lupus standardized for 8% lupulinum.

Safety

No known safety issues.

Interactions

May increase the sedative effects of sedative medications and alcohol.

References

1. Kings American Dispensatory 1898 available online at Henriette's Herbal Homepage [online] at http://www.henriettesherbal.com/eclectic/kings/index.html
2. The British Pharmaceutical Codex 1907 available online at Henriette's Herbal Homepage [online] at http://www.henriettesherbal.com/eclectic/bpc1911/index.html
3. Lupulinum. Kings American Dispensary. Henriette's Herbal Homepage. [online] at http://www.henriettesherbal.com/eclectic/kings/humulus_lupulin.html
4. Schiller H, Forster A, Vonhoff C, Hegger M, Biller A, Winterhoff H. Sedating effects of Humulus lupulus L. extracts. Phytomedicine. 2006;13(8):535-41. Epub 2006 Jul 24
5. Morin CM, Koetter U, Bastien C, Ware JC, Wooten V. Valerian-hops combination and diphenhydramine for treating insomnia: a randomized placebo-controlled clinical trial. Sleep. 2005;28(11):1465-71
6. Dimpfel W, Suter A. Sleep improving effects of a single dose administration of a valerian/hops fluid extract - a double blind, randomized, placebo-controlled sleep-EEG study in a parallel design using electrohypnograms. Eur J Med Res. 2008 May;13(5):200-4
7. Milligan SR, Kalita JC, Heyerick A, Rong H, De Cooman L, De Keukeleire D. Identification of a potent phytoestrogen in hops (Humulus lupulus L.) and beer. J Clin Endocrinol Metab. 1999;84(6):2249-52

Idebenone

Other names

2-(10-hydroxydecyl)-5,6-dimethoxy-3-methylcyclohexa-2,5-diene-1,4-dione
2,3-dimethoxy-5-methyl-6-(10-hydroxydecyl)-1,4-benzoquinone

Star rating

2

What is it?

Idebenone is a synthetic analogue of coenzyme Q which acts as a free radical scavenger and protects the mitochondrial membrane against lipid peroxidation. It has an anti-oxidant potency similar to vitamin E (1).

Claimed benefits

Improves focus, concentration and learning.
Improves energy production.

Mode of Action

The mode of action for improving focus and concentration is unknown but studies suggest its anti free radical action protects against nerve cell damage and corrects neurotransmitter defects (2).

Idebenone may improve energy production by improving mitochondrial respiratory chain function and energy production (3).

Effectiveness

Idebenone has been shown in a number of small studies to have a moderate benefit in older people suffering from cognitive decline and dementia, similar in effect to the nootropic compound oxiracetam (4).

One small study has also shown that idebenone can protect the brain of healthy young males against damage caused by hypoxia (5).

However there is currently no evidence available showing that idebenone can improve brain function in a way that improves sporting performance.

In a study on mice who had a genetic mutation which mimics the human disease muscular dystrophy, idebenone did appear able to improve energy production. The mice given idebenone were able to run faster than mice who were given a placebo (3). However in a human study, children with Friedrich's ataxia (an inherited disease affecting nerves and muscles) had no benefit to their exercise capacity from six months treatment with idebenone (6).

There is no current evidence that idebenone could improve sporting performance or exercise capacity in healthy humans.

Commonly used dosages

Idebenone is usually included as part of a proprietary formulation in commercial sport supplement preparations with the exact quantity of the substance not listed in the ingredients.

It is possible to buy idebenone as a stand alone supplement

both in capsules and as a free powder.

In the study mentioned above showing a protective effect in brains of healthy young males they were given 300mg, 3x/day.

Absorption of idebenone is greater (up to 5 x greater) if it is taken after meals (7).

Safety

No known safety issues.

Interactions

None known.

References

1. Mordente A, Martorana GE, Minotti G, Giardina B. Antioxidant properties of 2,3-dimethoxy-5-methyl-6-(10-hydroxydecyl)-1,4-benzoquinone (idebenone). Chem Res Toxicol. 1998;11(1):54-63
2. Gillis JC, Benefield P, McTavish D. Idebenone. A review of its pharmacodynamic and pharmacokinetic properties, and therapeutic use in age-related cognitive disorders. Drugs Aging. 1994;5(2):133-52
3. Buyse GM, Van der Mieren G, Erb M, D'hooge J, Herijgers P, Verbeken E *et al.* Long-term blinded placebo-controlled study of SNT-MC17/idebenone in the dystrophin deficient mdx mouse: cardiac protection and improved exercise performance. Eur Heart J. 2009;30(1):116-24. Epub 2008 Sep 10
4. Gillis JC, Benefield P, McTavish D. Idebenone. A review of its pharmacodynamic and pharmacokinetic properties,

and therapeutic use in age-related cognitive disorders.
Drugs Aging. 1994;5(2):133-52

5. Schaffler K, Hadler D, Stark M. Dose-effect relationship of idebenone in an experimental cerebral deficit model. Pilot study in healthy young volunteers with piracetam as reference drug. Arzneimittelforschung. 1998;48(7):720-6

6. Drinkard BE, Keyser RE, Paul SM, Arena R, Plehn JF *et al*. Exercise capacity and idebenone intervention in children and adolescents with Friedreich ataxia. Arch Phys Med Rehabil. 2010;91(7):1044-50

7. Kutz K, Drewe J, Vankan P. Pharmacokinetic properties and metabolism of idebenone. J Neurol. 2009;256 Suppl 1:31-5

Jojoba

Other names

Deer nut
Goat nut
Jojoba Meal
Pig nut
Simmondsia chinensis

Star rating

2

What is it?

A shrub of the Simmondsiaceae family which grows in the deserts of Arizona, California and Mexico.

The seeds of jojoba are approximately 50% composed of wax esters which are commonly used in the manufacture of cosmetics for their emollient properties. The remaining part of the seed is known as defatted jojoba meal and it is this part which is usually included in sport supplements (1).

Claimed benefits

Weight loss.

Mode of Action

Defatted jojoba meal contains the cyanoglucosides simmondsin and simmondsin ferrulate which have been shown in animal studies to reduce food intake and body weight (1).

It seems to achieve this by increasing satiety (feeling of fullness after eating food) by acting on the vagal nerve (2).

Effectiveness

Jojoba meal has been shown to decrease food intake and reduce weight in chickens, rats and dogs (1) (2) (3) but no studies have been carried out in humans.

Commonly used dosages

Jojoba is usually included as part of a proprietary formulation in commercial sport supplement preparations with the exact quantity of the substance not listed in the ingredients.

It is not possible to buy jojoba meal as a stand-alone supplement.

Safety

There is uncertainty in the scientific literature regarding the safety of simmondsin, the active compound in jojoba meal. In some studies rats fed simmondsin developed bone marrow suppression and anemia, especially at higher doses (3) (4). Given this it would seem sensible to avoid consuming jojoba containing supplements until further information is available regarding its safety.

Interactions

None known.

References

1. Hawthorne AJ, Butterwick RF. The satiating effect of a diet containing jojoba meal (Simmondsia chinensis) in dogs. J Nutr. 1998;128(12 Suppl):2669S-2670S
2. Flo G, Van Boven M, Vermaut S, Daenens P, Decuypere E, Cokelaere M. The vagus nerve is involved in the anorexigenic effect of simmondsin in the rat. Appetite. 2000;34(2):147-51
3. Boozer CN, Herron AJ. Simmondsin for weight loss in rats. Int J Obes (Lond). 2006;30(7):1143-8. Epub 2006 Feb 7
4. York DA, Singer L, Oliver J, Abbott TP, Bray GA. The detrimental effect of simmondsin on food intake and body weight of rats. Ind Crops Prod 2000;12(3):183-192

Methoxyisoflavone

Other names

5-Methyl-7-Methoxy-Isoflavone
7 methoxy
7-methoxy-3-phenyl-4H-chromen-4-one
7-methoxyisoflavone
Methoxyflavone

Star rating

1

What is it?

An artificially developed compound which was patented by the Hungarian pharmaceutical company Chinoin in 1977 along with various other similar compounds (1) (2). It is based on the structure of naturally occurring plant flavones but does not itself appear to exist naturally in plants.

Claimed benefits

Anabolic action and anti-catabolic action.

Mode of Action

No specific mode of action was described in the patent although it stated that the compounds increased nitrogen retention. The patent claimed that the compounds had an anabolic effect with no androgenic or estrogenic effect. The anti-catabolic effect was stated to be due to the ability of the compounds to suppress the catabolic effect of cortisone.

Effectiveness

According to the patent chickens fed methoxyisoflavone for periods up to 8 weeks had weight gains of up to 10%. A related compund 7-isopropoxy-isoflavone (which according to the patent was less anabolic than methoxyisoflavone) was claimed to be stronger than equivalent doses of anabolic steroids, although which anabolic steroids were tested was not revealed. 7-isopropoxy-isoflavone was tested on underweight human patients recovering from illness and found to increase weight by 2-3kg over a period of several weeks. However none of this research was submitted for publication in any scientific journal.

For unknown reasons Chinoin did not further develop any of their patented compounds and the patent lapsed after twenty years. When this happened various supplement companies began marketing it as a sport supplement. Scientific studies supporting its effectiveness were still lacking in the scientific literature until the supplement manufacturer Biotest sponsored a study in 2001 (3). This study claimed that of the seven males taking 800mg methoxyisoflavone for 8 weeks, increases in lean mass and reductions in body fat were observed compared to placebo. However this study was only published as an abstract in a supplement to the journal making it difficult to fully evaluate.

A larger randomised double blind study carried out in 2006, which was fully published, failed to find any benefit from methoxyisoflavone supplementation at 800mg per day for 8 weeks. No changes in anabolic/catabolic status were observed (4).

In summary, despite the promising claims of the original patent there remains virtually no evidence in support of methoxyisoflavone over 30 years later.

As a further comment, the original patent registered methoxyisoflavone for use in animal feeds. Marketing material for many sports supplements claim that it has been used for this purpose for many years to increase the weight of livestock. I have been unable to find any evidence at all that methoxyisoflavone has ever been used as an additive to animal feed or for veterinary purposes.

Commonly used dosages

Methoxyisoflavone is usually included as part of a proprietary formulation in commercial sport supplement preparations with the exact quantity of the substance not listed in the ingredients.

It is not usually sold as a stand alone supplement.

Safety

No known safety issues.

Interactions

None known.

References

1. Free Patents Online, United States Patent 4163746, Metabolic 5-methyl-isoflavone-derivatives, process for the preparation thereof and compositions containing the same [online] at http://www.freepatentsonline.com/4163746.html
2. Free Patents Online, United States Patent 3949085, Anabolic-weight-gain promoting compositions containing isoflavone derivatives and method using same

[online] at
http://www.freepatentsonline.com/3949085.html

3. Incledon T. The Effects of 5-Methyl-7-Methoxyisoflavone on Body Composition and Performance in College-Aged Men. Med Sci Sports Exer. 2001;33(5 suppl):S338 [abstract]

4. Wilborn CD, Taylor LW, Campbell BI, Kerksick C, Rasmussen CJ *et al*. Effects of methoxyisoflavone, ecdysterone, and sulfo-polysaccharide supplementation on training adaptations in resistance-trained males. J Int Soc Sports Nutr. 2006;3:19-27

Micellar Casein

Other names

Phosphocasein

Star rating

5

What is it?

A protein derived from milk.

Milk contains 3.3% protein containing all 8 essential amino acids. This protein is actually composed of two kinds of protein 82% casein and 18% whey. Both of these in turn are made up of various components. Whey is composed of about 50% ß-lactoglobulin, 20% α-lactalbumin and the balance made up of blood serum albumin, lactoferrin, transferrin, various immunoglobulins and other minor proteins. Casein is composed of 4 different caseins which all have their own amino acid structure; α-s1, α-s2 , ß, and kappa-casein. These caseins naturally bind together to form small spherical units called "micelles".

Casein micelles keep the protein in solution in water and are very stable. They are not affected by heat (unlike whey which can be denatured by high temperature) and can be dried and reconstituted etc. without losing their structure (1).

After the fat is removed from milk to leave skimmed milk, this can be subjected to various further processes to extract its casein and whey protein content.

Caseinates are obtained by addition of an acid to the milk. This causes the micelles of casein to precipitate or fall out of solution at pH 4.6. The resulting acid casein is collected and then the acid neutralized by addition of an alkali such as calcium, sodium or potassium thus producing calcium caseinate or sodium caseinate etc. Due to the chemical processing involved which can alter the structure and properties of the protein (and the taste), caseinates are generally considered an inferior protein source to micellar casein or whey protein.

Other methods rely on filtration to extract the protein which leaves its structure and properties intact.

Ultrafiltration removes the lactose (milk carbohydrate content) from the milk leaving behind a milk protein concentrate (MPC) which contains the same proportions of micellar casein and whey as natural milk, i.e. 82% casein and 18% whey.

The other method is microfiltration. Microfiltration is capable of separating the casein and whey constituents to produce either pure micellar casein or whey. Microfiltered casein may sometimes then undergo diafiltration to further increase its purity (2).

Many micellar casein products on sale are in fact ultrafiltered MPC and thus only actually contain 82% micellar casein. Whether it is worth paying extra for a microfiltered protein containing a few more percent of micellar casein will be a matter of personal choice and budget. Brands can also be seen which combine micellar casein with the inferior caseinate.

Claimed benefits

A slow release protein which inhibits muscle breakdown for long periods of time, especially useful when the time between meals is prolonged such as at night while sleeping.

Mode of Action

Micellar casein is digested very slowly and has a long transit time through the gastrointestinal tract. There appear to be two main reasons for this.

Firstly, in the acidic environment of the stomach, micellar casein precipitates out of solution (clots) and forms a solid gel like substance in the stomach. Solids empty from the stomach much more slowly than liquids. The micellar casein gel is partially digested by peptic acid in the stomach and then released slowly into the intestine where it is further digested by pancreatic enzymes and absorbed in the upper part of the small intestine. Whey protein on the other hand remains soluble in the stomach and exits quickly undigested in liquid form. It then undergoes digestion by pancreatic enzymes and is absorbed in the lower part of the small intestine (3) (4).

Secondly, β-casein contains opioid like peptides called β-casomorphins. These are released during the digestion of casein and directly interact with gut opioid receptors, inhibiting smooth muscle contractility in the gut and slowing gastrointestinal transit time (5).

Opioid like peptides have also been isolated from α-casein (6) and kappa-casein (7).

Effectiveness

The first and most famous study which looked at the different effects of whey protein versus micellar casein was that carried out by Yves Boirie *et al*. (8) in 1997. They gave 16 volunteers either a whey or casein meal and measured the effects.

In summary they found that in the first two hours after ingestion whey protein increased net protein synthesis by 68% while casein increased it by 31%. However, whey did not inhibit whole body protein breakdown at all, while casein inhibited protein breakdown by 34% for 7 hours. Casein caused blood plasma amino acid concentrations to remain above baseline after 5 hours while with whey they had dropped below baseline at 5 hours.

These findings have been replicated in several subsequent studies, all confirming that slow release proteins such as micellar casein lead to greater whole body net protein increases than fast release proteins (9) (10) (11) (12).

In terms of "real world results" in a study (13) involving overweight policemen given either whey or casein while dieting and undertaking a resistance exercise program for 12 weeks, both groups lost equal amounts of fat while the increase in lean mass (muscle) was 100% greater for the casein group compared to the whey group (+ 4kg for casein versus + 2kg for whey). Strength increases were 30% higher for the casein group (+ 59% versus +29% for whey). These differences being attributed to improved nitrogen retention and overall anti-catabolic effects caused by the casein.

Commonly used dosages

Daily protein intakes will vary considerably between individuals according to bodyweight and training goals. For bodybuilders and other sports people undergoing strenuous exercise regimes it is recommended to consume 2-3g of protein per kg of bodyweight.

Safety

No known safety issues.

Interactions

None known.

References

1. Cornell University, Milk Protein [online] at http://www.milkfacts.info/Milk%20Composition/protein.htm
2. Tamime AY. Dairy powders and concentrated milk products. Chichester, Wiley-Blackwell; 2009
3. Mahé S, Roos N, Benamouzig R, Davin L, Luengo C *et al.* Gastrojejunal kinetics and the digestion of [15N]beta-lactoglobulin and casein in humans: the influence of the nature and quantity of the protein. Am J Clin Nutr. 1996;63(4):546-52
4. Mahé S, Huneau JF, Marteau P, Thuillier F, Tomé D. Gastroileal nitrogen and electrolyte movements after

bovine milk ingestion in humans. Am J Clin Nutr. 1992;56(2):410-6

5. Daniel H, Vohwinkel M, Rehner G. Effect of casein and beta-casomorphins on gastrointestinal motility in rats. J Nutr. 1990;120(3):252-7

6. Loukas S, Varoucha D, Zioudrou C, Streaty RA, Klee WA. Opioid activities and structures of alpha-casein-derived exorphins. Biochemistry. 1983 Sep;22(19):4567-73

7. Stan EIa, Groĭsman SD, Krasil'shchikov KB, Chernikov MP. [Effect of kappa-casein glycomacropeptide on gastrointestinal motility in dogs] [Article in Russian] Biull Eksp Biol Med. 1983;96(7):10-2

8. Boirie Y, Dangin M, Gachon P, Vasson MP, Maubois JL, Beaufrère B. Slow and fast dietary proteins differently modulate postprandial protein accretion. Proc Natl Acad Sci U S A. 1997;94(26):14930-5

9. Dangin M, Boirie Y, Garcia-Rodenas C, Gachon P, Fauquant J *et al.* The digestion rate of protein is an independent regulating factor of postprandial protein retention. Am J Physiol Endocrinol Metab. 2001;280(2):E340-8

10. Dangin M, Boirie Y, Guillet C, Beaufrère B. Influence of the protein digestion rate on protein turnover in young and elderly subjects. J Nutr. 2002;132(10):3228S-33S

11. Deglaire A, Fromentin C, Fouillet H, Airinei G, Gaudichon C *et al.* Hydrolyzed dietary casein as compared with the intact protein reduces postprandial peripheral, but not whole-body, uptake of nitrogen in humans. Am J Clin Nutr. 2009;90(4):1011-22. Epub 2009 Aug 19

12. Lacroix M, Bos C, Léonil J, Airinei G, Luengo C *et al.* Compared with casein or total milk protein, digestion of milk soluble proteins is too rapid to sustain the anabolic postprandial amino acid requirement. Am J Clin Nutr. 2006;84(5):1070-9

13. Demling RH, DeSanti L. Effect of a hypocaloric diet, increased protein intake and resistance training on lean mass gains and fat mass loss in overweight police officers. Ann Nutr Metab. 2000;44(1):21-9

Milk Thistle

Other names

Marian Thistle
Silibinin
Silybin
Silybum
Silybum marianum
Silymarin
St. Mary Thistle

Star rating

4

What is it?

A flowering plant of the Asteraceae family native to North Africa the Middle East and the Mediterranean regions of Europe. It has a long tradition of use in traditional herbal medicine for treating jaundice and other ailments of the liver.

Claimed benefits

Hepatoprotective, that is it protects the liver against stress and damage caused by other substances. Sports people may use it to protect the liver from the toxic effects of other compounds used to enhance performance such as anabolic steroids, pro-hormones or other compounds.

Mode of Action

The fruit of milk thistle is rich in compounds such as sterols, flavonoids and flavolignans. A group of flavolignans referred to as silymarin is the main active constituent of the plant responsible for the hepatoprotective effects. Silymarin itself is composed mainly of silibinin (approximately 50-70%), silichristin, silidianin and smaller amounts of various other compounds (1) (2).

Of these silibinin is the most important since silichristin is not absorbed well in the gastrointestinal tract and silidianin is metabolized very quickly (3).

How silymarin protects the liver is not fully understood but seems to involve several distinct mechanisms. Silymarin is a potent antioxidant and free radical scavenger, it inhibits nitric oxide production and lipid peroxidation, which can damage cell membranes, and binds toxic free iron (2).

In addition, silymarin can prevent toxins from entering cells by competing with them for receptor sites on the cell membrane and help damaged liver cells regenerate by increasing protein synthesis (3).

Finally, silymarin is able to prevent TNF (Tumor Necrosis Factor) induced inflammation and cell destruction (4).

Effectiveness

It is difficult to assess the effectiveness of milk thistle in protecting the liver since there are so many mechanisms of liver injury and milk thistle may be effective in protecting against some mechanisms but be less effective against others. In general terms, most of the studies on milk thistle have looked at 4 major mechanisms of damage which are alcoholic hepatitis, viral hepatitis, poisoning by death cap mushroom (Amanita phalloides), and acute toxicity caused by various other drugs and poisons.

Of these, acute toxicity caused by drugs and poisoning by death cap mushroom are the most relevant to our discussion since they most closely resemble the possible effects of performance enhancing agents such as anabolic steroids and pro-hormones on the livers of sports people.

I looked at 6 major reviews (conducted between 2001 and 2008) which analysed all the studies available on milk thistle. The conclusions of these reviews can be summarised as follows: milk thistle has very good evidence supporting its use as a treatment for death cap mushroom poisoning. Milk thistle is probably effective at improving markers of liver damage in alcoholic cirrhosis, although there is less evidence it improves long term outcomes. There is little evidence that milk thistle has any beneficial effect in treatment of viral hepatitis (5) (6) (7) (8) (9) (10).

Regarding evidence for the effects of milk thistle in cases of acute poisoning by drugs or other compounds, human studies are difficult to find due to the obvious ethical problems of using poisoned individuals to study experimental treatments. However there is one study in which industrial workers found to have abnormal liver function tests after being exposed to toluene and/or xylene vapours for 5-20 years were given milk thistle extract 3 times daily (Legalon® formulation – see below under commonly used dosages for information regarding Legalon®). After 30 days the liver function tests of all the workers improved (11).

In other studies carried out on animals, milk thistle has been been shown to protect against acute poisoning caused by ethanol (12) cyclosporin (13) phalloidin (14) tetracycline (15) arsenic (16) and carbon tetrachloride (17).

In conclusion while there is no specific evidence for the hepatoprotective action of milk thistle against the effects of anabolic steroids or pro-hormones, the best evidence for the use of milk thistle shows it to be effective in similar situations of acute toxicity against a wide range of other hepato-toxins. In particular there is good human evidence that milk thistle is effective for the treatment of death cap mushroom poisoning.

Commonly used dosages

Milk thistle is usually sold as a stand alone product of milk thistle extract in doses ranging from 100mg to 350mg. Some brands specifically state that they are standardized to contain a certain percentage of silymarin with amounts of 70-80% being common.

It should be noted that the original standardized milk thistle extract of 70 percent silymarin was produced by a German company called Madaus. Madaus produce a pharmaceutical quality milk thistle product called Legalon® which is sold in tablets containing 70 or 140 milligrams of silymarin and which can be taken in a dose of one to two tablets three times a day. Legalon® is also available in an intravenous form for use in treatment of death cap mushroom poisoning.

Legalon® has been shown to have superior release and bioavailability of silibinin than many other milk thistle preparations (3) and is sold in the USA under the name Thisilyn® by the company Nature's Way.

Madaus outsources production of its crude silymarin to an Italian company called Indena. Indena has itself developed a form of purified silibinin complexed with phosphatidylcholine which has been shown to have even greater bioavailabilty up to 10 times greater than other oral preparations (3). This form of silibinin is called IdB 1016 or Silipide® and is marketed in the USA by Indena USA Inc. under the tradename Siliphos® (18).

Safety

No known safety issues.

Interactions

Silibinin has been shown to increase the bioavailability of tamoxifen in rats. It is unknown if it has similar effects in humans (19).

References

1. Barnes J, Anderson LA, Phillipson JD. Herbal Medicines. 3rd ed. London: Pharmaceutical Press; 2007
2. Venkataramanan R, Ramachandran V, Komoroski BJ, Zhang S, Schiff PL, Strom SC. Milk thistle, a herbal supplement, decreases the activity of CYP3A4 and uridine diphosphoglucuronosyl transferase in human hepatocyte cultures. Drug Metab Dispos. 2000;28(11):1270-3
3. National Library of Medicine, Agency for Healthcare Research and Quality, AHRQ Evidence Reports, Milk Thistle: Effects on Liver Disease and Cirrhosis and Clinical Adverse Effects [online] at http://www.ncbi.nlm.nih.gov/bookshelf/br.fcgi?book=er ta21&part=A30173#A30175

4. Manna SK, Mukhopadhyay A, Van NT, Aggarwal BB. Silymarin suppresses TNF-induced activation of NF-kappa B, c-Jun N-terminal kinase, and apoptosis. J Immunol. 1999;163(12):6800-9

5. Wellington K, Jarvis B. Silymarin: a review of its clinical properties in the management of hepatic disorders. BioDrugs. 2001;15(7):465-89

6. Saller R, Meier R, Brignoli R. The use of silymarin in the treatment of liver diseases. Drugs. 2001;61(14):2035-63

7. Saller R, Brignoli R, Melzer J, Meier R. An updated systematic review with meta-analysis for the clinical evidence of silymarin. Forsch Komplementmed. 2008;15(1):9-20

8. Mayer KE, Myers RP, Lee SS. Silymarin treatment of viral hepatitis: a systematic review. J Viral Hepat. 2005;12(6):559-67

9. Tamayo C, Diamond S. Review of clinical trials evaluating safety and efficacy of milk thistle (Silybum marianum [L.] Gaertn.). Integr Cancer Ther. 2007;6(2):146-57

10. Rambaldi A, Jacobs BP, Gluud C. Milk thistle for alcoholic and/or hepatitis B or C virus liver diseases. Cochrane Database Syst Rev. 2007;(4):CD003620

11. Szilárd S, Szentgyörgyi D, Demeter I. Protective effect of Legalon in workers exposed to organic solvents. Acta Med Hung. 1988;45(2):249-56

12. Song Z, Deaciuc I, Song M, Lee DY, Liu Y *et al.* Silymarin protects against acute ethanol-induced hepatotoxicity in mice. Alcohol Clin Exp Res. 2006;30(3):407-13

13. Zima T, Kameníková L, Janebová M, Buchar E, Crkovská J, Tesar V. The effect of silibinin on experimental cyclosporine nephrotoxicity. Ren Fail. 1998;20(3):471-9

14. Tuchweber B, Sieck R, Trost W. Prevention of silybin of phalloidin-induced acute hepatoxicity. Toxicol Appl Pharmacol. 1979;51(2):265-75

15. Porokhniak LA, Drogovoz SM, Rogozhin BA. [Action of hepatoprotective agents in a tetracycline lesion of the liver] [Article in Russian] Antibiot Med Biotekhnol. 1987;32(4):282-5
16. Jain A, Yadav A, Bozhkov AI, Padalko VI, Flora SJ. Therapeutic efficacy of silymarin and naringenin in reducing arsenic-induced hepatic damage in young rats. Ecotoxicol Environ Saf. 2010 Aug 17. [Epub ahead of print]
17. Kim SH, Cheon HJ, Yun N, Oh ST, Shin E *et al.* Protective effect of a mixture of Aloe vera and Silybum marianum against carbon tetrachloride-induced acute hepatotoxicity and liver fibrosis. J Pharmacol Sci. 2009;109(1):119-27
18. Blumenthal M, Goldberg A, Kunz T. The ABC Clinical Guide to Herbs. New York: Thieme Medical Publishers Inc; 2003
19. Kim CS, Choi SJ, Park CY, Li C, Choi JS. Effects of silybinin on the pharmacokinetics of tamoxifen and its active metabolite, 4-hydroxytamoxifen in rats. Anticancer Res. 2010;30(1):79-85

Mucuna pruriens

Other names

Carpopogon pruriens
Cowhage
Cow-Itch Plant
Dolichos pruriens
Mucuna aterrima
Mucuna cochinchinensis
Mucuna prurita
Stizolobium aterrimum
Stizolobium pruriens
Velvet Bean

Star rating

4

What is it?

A climbing vine of the Fabaceae family which grows in tropical regions particularly South America, India, Africa and the West Indies. It has a long tradition of use in traditional and Ayurvedic medicine as an aphrodisiac, treatment for impotence and male infertility, Parkinson's disease and for various other ailments.

Claimed benefits

Mucuna pruriens is claimed to increase levels of testosterone and growth hormone causing an anabolic action and decreased levels of fat tissue.

Mode of Action

To increase testosterone levels mucuna pruriens is thought to act on the pituitary gland, stimulating it to release more luteinizing hormone which acts on the Leydig cells in the testes stimulating them to produce more testosterone (1). Exactly how it does this is unknown.

To increase levels of growth hormone (GH) mucuna pruriens acts by increasing levels of the hormone dopamine which is believed to stimulate the hypothalamus in the brain to release more Growth Hormone Releasing Hormone (GHRH) which causes the pituitary gland to release more GH (2).

Mucuna pruriens is able to increase dopamine levels since it contains between 3-6% of levodopa (L-dopa) (3) (4) which is converted in the brain by the enzyme L-aromatic amino acid decarboxylase to produce dopamine.

Effectiveness

There is only one human study (1) which has tested the ability of mucuna pruriens to increase testosterone levels which was carried out on 75 infertile men who had low initial testosterone levels compared to healthy controls. These men experienced an increase in testosterone levels from 17-39% after supplementing with 5g/day of mucuna pruriens powder for 3 months. Unfortunately the healthy controls were not also given the mucuna pruriens in this study so we are unable to assess its effect in healthy men.

The ability of mucuna pruriens to increase GH levels has not been directly tested in humans however its mechanism of action can be considered proved since the ability of L-dopa consumed orally has been demonstrated to cause considerable increases in GH levels in normal healthy humans. From a baseline of plasma GH level of less than 1ng/mL, 500mg of L-dopa taken orally has been seen to increase GH levels up to 24ng/mL (5) (6) (7) (8). The GH begins to rise after 30 minutes and begins to slowly decline at 2 hours after consumption of L-dopa (compared to a half life of 30-40 minutes for GH given intravenously or 3-4 hours if given subcutaneously).

While like for like comparisons are hard to make the increase in plasma GH of up to 24ng/ml caused by administration of L-dopa can be compared to information given by Lilly in the prescribing information for Humatrope® an artificially produced GH. This states that subcutaneous administration of 0.1mg/kg of Humatrope® (equivalent to 19iu of GH for a 70kg man) produces a maximum plasma GH of 63ng/mL.

The effects of lower amounts of L-dopa to the standard 500mg used in these studies is unknown but the release of GH may be dose dependent and smaller amounts of L-dopa would stimulate proportionally smaller amounts of GH.

In summary while there is only one study demonstrating that mucuna pruriens increases testosterone levels, the fact that L-dopa stimulates growth hormone release can be considered proved.

Commonly used dosages

Mucuna pruriens is usually included as part of a proprietary formulation in commercial sport supplement preparations with the exact quantity of the substance not listed in the ingredients. Extracts of mucuna pruriens in sport supplements are usually standardized to contain around 15% L-dopa.

Mucuna pruriens is also available as a stand alone product.

Capsules of 800mg extract standardized to 15% and containing 120mg L-dopa are available.

Bioavailability of L-dopa from mucuna pruriens has been shown to be equivalent to pharmaceutical L-dopa used in the treatment of Parkinson's disease (9) and in fact promising trials have been carried out suggesting mucuna pruriens may be a superior treatment for Parkinson's than pharmaceutically produced L-dopa (10).

Safety

In trials, people taking mucuna pruriens containing up to 1000mg of L-dopa reported adverse events such as mild nausea, mild gastric pain and dizziness (10).

However any of the side effects of the prescription medicine L-dopa are theoretically possible with mucuna pruriens intake. These include loss of appetite, nausea and vomiting, itching, insomnia, involuntary movements, tachycardia, reddish discoloration of urine, depression and psychosis. Also sudden onset of daytime sleepiness has been reported so care should be exercised if driving or operating machinery. Most of these have not been reported with mucuna pruriens use, however there is one report of psychosis associated with mucuna pruriens intake (11).

Interactions

Similarly, any of the known interactions of prescription L-dopa are theoretically possible with mucuna pruriens. Anyone taking any prescription medication should consult with their doctor before taking mucuna pruriens.

L-dopa interacts with a wide range of medications, some of the more serious interactions are -

- Enhanced hypotensive effect with antihypotensives such as ACE inhibitors, alpha blockers, beta blockers, calcium channel blockers and methyldopa.

- Increased risk of arrythmias with general anesthetics.

- Risk of hypertensive crisis when taken with MAOIs

References

1. Shukla KK, Mahdi AA, Ahmad MK, Shankhwar SN, Rajender S, Jaiswar SP. Mucuna pruriens improves male fertility by its action on the hypothalamus-pituitary-gonadal axis. Fertil Steril. 2009;92(6):1934-40. Epub 2008 Oct 29

2. Mitsuhashi S, Yamasaki R, Miyazaki S, Saito H, Saito S. [Effect of oral administration of L-dopa on the plasma levels of growth hormone-releasing hormone (GHRH) in normal subjects and patients with various endocrine and metabolic diseases] [Article in Japanese] Nippon Naibunpi Gakkai Zasshi. 1987;63(8):934-46

3. No authors listed. An alternative medicine treatment for Parkinson's disease: results of a multicenter clinical trial. HP-200 in Parkinson's Disease Study Group. J Altern Complement Med. 1995;1(3):249-55

4. Infante ME, Perez AM, Simao MR, Manda F, Baquete EF *et al.* Outbreak of acute toxic psychosis attributed to Mucuna pruriens. Lancet. 1990;336(8723):1129

5. Tapanainen P, Knip M, Lautala P, Leppäluoto J. Variable plasma growth hormone (GH)-releasing hormone and GH responses to clonidine, L-dopa, and insulin in normal men. J Clin Endocrinol Metab. 1988;67(4):845-9

6. Mitsuhashi S, Yamasaki R, Miyazaki S, Saito H, Saito S. [Effect of oral administration of L-dopa on the plasma levels of growth hormone-releasing hormone (GHRH) in normal subjects and patients with various endocrine and

metabolic diseases] [Article in Japanese] Nippon Naibunpi Gakkai Zasshi. 1987;63(8):934-46

7. Verde G, Oppizzi G, Colussi G, Cremascoli G, Botalla L *et al.* Effect of dopamine infusion on plasma levels of growth hormone in normal subjects and in agromegalic patients. Clin Endocrinol (Oxf). 1976;5(4):419-23

8. Chihara K, Kashio Y, Kita T, Okimura Y, Kaji H *et al.* L-dopa stimulates release of hypothalamic growth hormone-releasing hormone in humans. J Clin Endocrinol Metab. 1986;62(3):466-73

9. Mahajani SS, Doshi VJ, Parikh KM, Manyam BV. Bioavailability of L-DOPA from HP-200—a Formulation of Seed Powder of Mucuna pruriens (Bak): a Pharmacokinetic and Pharmacodynamic Study. Phytother Res 1996;10(3):254-256

10. Katzenschlager R, Evans A, Manson A, Patsalos PN, Ratnaraj N *et al.* Mucuna pruriens in Parkinson's disease: a double blind clinical and pharmacological study. J Neurol Neurosurg Psychiatry. 2004;75(12):1672-7

11. Infante ME, Perez AM, Simao MR, Manda F, Baquete EF *et al.* Outbreak of acute toxic psychosis attributed to Mucuna pruriens. Lancet. 1990;336(8723):1129

Naringin

Other names

(2S)-7-[(2S,3R,4S,5S,6R)-4,5-dihydroxy-6-(hydroxymethyl)-
3-[(2S,3R,4R,   5R,6S)-3,4,5-trihydroxy-6-methyloxan-2-
yl]oxyoxan-2-yl]oxy-5-hydroxy-2-(4-   hydroxyphenyl)-2,3-
dihydrochromen-4-one
4',5,7-trihydroxyflavanone 7-rhamnoglucoside
4'5-diOH-Flavone-7-rhgluc
7-[[2-O-(6-Deoxy-α-L-mannopyranosyl)-β-D-
glucopyranosyl]oxy]-2,3-dihydro-5-hydroxy-2-(4-
hydroxyphenyl)-4H-1-benzopyran-4-one
Aurantiin
Naringenin-7-rhamnoglucoside
Naringoside

Star rating

2

What is it?

The major flavonoid glycoside found in grapefruit and it is
the substance which gives grapefruit its bitter taste. After
consumption naringin is converted to naringenin in the
intestine.

Claimed benefits

Increases the half life of caffeine prolonging its time in the
human system before it is broken down and hence
prolonging its effect.

This is of use to sports people taking caffeine or caffeine
containing supplements to enhance performance.

Mode of Action

It is claimed that naringin inhibits the cytochrome P450 enzyme CYP1A2 in the liver. CYP1A2 is the enzyme responsible for the breakdown of caffeine in the human body.

Effectiveness

The discovery that grapefruit juice can affect the metabolism of drugs and increase their bioavailability was made by accident in 1989 during a study into the effects of alcohol on the blood pressure drug felodipine. Grapefruit juice was given to hide the taste of the alcohol and researchers noticed that it markedly increased blood levels of the drug. Subsequent investigations revealed that grapefruit juice down-regulates the cytochrome P450 enzyme CYP3A4 present in the intestines and which breaks down many drugs before they are absorbed (1).

It was subsequently discovered that grapefruit juice also inhibits CYP1A2 and can increase the half life of caffeine *in vivo* in humans by 31% (2).

In vitro tests initially indicated that the active principle in grapefruit juice responsible for these effects was naringin (1) however subsequent studies have revealed that naringin does not make a major contribution to inhibiting P450 enzymes and that other constituents are primarily responsible (3) with the compound bergapten being the most potent inhibitor (4).

A further *in vivo* study found that naringin alone has no affect on caffeine pharmacokinetics in humans (5).

In summary the use of naringin is not justified and it would

273

be better to drink grapefruit juice in order to inhibit the metabolism of caffeine until new supplements based on the true main active constituents are available on the market.

Note: Effect of grapefruit juice on estrogen levels –

Estrogen is also metabolized by CYP3A4 and so estrogen levels can be increased by grapefruit. Post menopausal women who consume ¼ grapefruit or more per day have been found to have higher estrogen levels (estradiol 10% higher and estrone 30% higher) than women who do not consume grapefruit (6). This leads to a 25-30% increased breast cancer risk for post menopausal women (7).

Therefore I recommend that sports people who wish to maintain low levels of estrogen completely avoid grapefruit juice.

Commonly used dosages

Naringin is usually included as part of a proprietary formulation in commercial sport supplement preparations with the exact quantity of the substance not listed in the ingredients.

It is not usually sold as a stand alone supplement.

Safety

No known safety issues.

Interactions

While it is now believed that naringin is not the main compound in grapefuit juice which affects the P450 enzymes and increases blood levels of many drugs, it may still have a small effect. Therefore it would be cautious to avoid taking naringin with any drug known to be affected by grapefruit, of which there are many. These include anti-arrhythmics, anti-malarials, anxiolytics, calcium channel blockers, ciclosporin, lipid regulating drugs, sildenafil, tadalafil, vardenafil and tacrolimus. Please consult your doctor if in any doubt.

References

1. Bailey DG, Malcolm J, Arnold O, Spence JD. Grapefruit juice-drug interactions. Br J Clin Pharmacol. 1998;46(2):101-10
2. Fuhr U, Klittich K, Staib AH. Inhibitory effect of grapefruit juice and its bitter principal, naringenin, on CYP1A2 dependent metabolism of caffeine in man. Br J Clin Pharmacol. 1993;35(4):431-6
3. Edwards DJ, Bernier SM. Naringin and naringenin are not the primary CYP3A inhibitors in grapefruit juice. Life Sci. 1996;59(13):1025-30
4. Ho PC, Saville DJ, Wanwimolruk S. Inhibition of human CYP3A4 activity by grapefruit flavonoids, furanocoumarins and related compounds. J Pharm Pharm Sci. 2001;4(3):217-27
5. Ballard TL, Halaweish FT, Stevermer CL, Agrawal P, Vukovich MD. Naringin does not alter caffeine pharmacokinetics, energy expenditure, or cardiovascular haemodynamics in humans following caffeine consumption. Clin Exp Pharmacol Physiol. 2006;33(4):310-4.
6. Monroe KR, Murphy SP, Henderson BE, Kolonel LN, Stanczyk FZ *et al.* Dietary fiber intake and endogenous serum hormone levels in naturally postmenopausal Mexican American women: the Multiethnic Cohort Study. Nutr Cancer. 2007;58(2):127-35
7. Monroe KR, Murphy SP, Kolonel LN, Pike MC. Prospective study of grapefruit intake and risk of breast

cancer in postmenopausal women: the Multiethnic Cohort Study. Br J Cancer. 2007;97(3):440-5. Epub 2007 Jul 10

Nettle

Other names

Divanillyltetrahydrofuran
Stinging nettle
Urtica dioica
Urtica urens

Star rating

3

What is it?

A common perennial plant of the family Urticaceae and usually considered a weed. Found throughout Europe and the United States it grows to about 3' or 4' tall and is well known for its hairy stems and leaves which can cause a painful burning rash if brought into contact with the skin.

Claimed benefits

Can increase levels of free testosterone and reduce levels of estrogen.

Mode of Action

97% of circulating testosterone is bound to circulating proteins produced in the liver. Most is bound to sex hormone binding globulin (SHBG) and a smaller amount is also bound to a protein called albumin. Only the 3% which is unbound (free testosterone) is available to act on tissues (1).

The roots of nettle contain various lignans which have been found to bind to SHBG. Once bound to a nettle lignan less SHBG is available to bind to testosterone hence the amount of free testosterone is increased.

The nettle root lignans which have been found to bind to SHBG are neoolivil, secoisolariciresinol, dehydrodiconiferyl alcohol, isolariciresinol and 3,4-divanillyltetrahydrofuran. Of these 3,4-divanillyltetrahydrofuran shows the highest binding affinity for SHBG (2) (3).

Testosterone is converted into estrogens by the enzyme aromatase. Various studies have shown that compounds present in nettle extract are able to inhibit the aromatase enzyme and prevent this conversion (4). Specific compounds identified include secoisolariciresinol, oleanolic and ursolic acid, (9Z,11E)-13-hydroxy-9,11-octadecadienoic acid, and 14-octacosanol which are weak to moderate inhibitors of aromatase (5).

A final minor activity of nettle is its ability to inhibit the enzyme 5-alpha-reductase and hence prevent the conversion of testosterone into DHT (4). However its activity is very weak, one study showed it was 40,000 times weaker than the prescription drug finasteride at inhibiting 5-alpha-reductase (6) so its effect on testosterone levels via this mechanism is likely to be negligible.

Effectiveness

In human studies the effect of nettle on SHBG and testosterone levels has been mixed. In two double blind studies a decrease in SHBG and 10% increase in testosterone levels was seen after taking 1200mg/day for 7 months in one study while in another study no effect was found after taking 600mg for 9 weeks.

In non double blind studies changes in SHBG and testosterone were also observed with doses up to 1200mg/day (4).

Regarding the ability of nettle to prevent estrogen production by inhibiting aromatase, while compounds in nettle have been identified as weak to moderate inhibitors of aromatase, tests have only been carried out *in vitro* so at the current time we do not know what effect these would have in humans. In addition these compounds are only found in very small quantities in nettle. Further testing needs to be done.

Finally it should be pointed out that particular types of nettle extract may be required in order to achieve the desired effects. Nettle extracts can be aqueous, ethanol extract or methanol extract. Most of the *in vivo* evidence for SHBG binding and increase in testosterone used a methanol extract with a strength of 5:1 extract. Anti-aromatase activity *in vitro* has been seen with both ethanol and methanol extracts. 5-alpha-reductase inhibition was seen only with a methanol extract while the ethanol extract had no effect (4).

Commonly used dosages

Nettle extract can be found in sport supplements in amounts from 150mg to 400mg. It is also available as a stand alone supplement typically in capsules of 500mg or as liquid extracts. Often it is hard to find manufacturers information regarding the type of extract or strength (ratio of plant to extract).

Safety

Nettle has been reported to cause gastrointestinal complaints and can induce abortion and affect the uterus so it should be avoided by pregnant women (7).

Interactions

Nettle may interact with diabetes and blood pressure medications (7). Consult your doctor before taking nettle if you take any prescription medication.

References

1. Marshall WJ, Bangert SK. Clinical Chemistry 5th Edition. Philadelphia, Elsevier Ltd; 2004
2. Schöttner M, Gansser D, Spiteller G. Lignans from the roots of Urtica dioica and their metabolites bind to human sex hormone binding globulin (SHBG). Planta Med. 1997;63(6):529-32
3. Schöttner M, Gansser D, Spiteller G. Interaction of lignans with human sex hormone binding globulin (SHBG). Z Naturforsch C. 1997;52(11-12):834-43
4. Chrubasik JE, Roufogalis BD, Wagner H, Chrubasik S. A comprehensive review on the stinging nettle effect and efficacy profiles. Part II: urticae radix. Phytomedicine. 2007;14(7-8):568-79. Epub 2007 May 16
5. Gansser D, Spiteller G. Aromatase inhibitors from Urtica dioica roots. Planta Med. 1995;61(2):138-40
6. Rhodes L, Primka RL, Berman C, Vergult G, Gabriel M, *et al.* Comparison of finasteride (proscar®), a 5α reductase inhibitor, and various commercial plant extracts in in vitro and in vivo 5α reductase inhibition. The Prostate 1993;22(1):43-51
7. Barnes J, Anderson LA, Phillipson JD. Herbal Medicines. 3rd ed. London: Pharmaceutical Press; 2007

Norvaline

Other names

L-norvaline
2-Aminovaleric acid
2-Aminopentanoic acid
Alpha-aminovaleric acid

Star rating

2

What is it?

A straight chain analogue of the branched chain amino acid valine. Although it is an amino acid it is not found in protein and is usually manufactured synthetically although it is produced naturally by certain bacteria such as *E.coli*, *Bacillus subtilis* and *Serratia marcescens* (1).

Claimed benefits

A vasodilator helping the user to achieve a "pump" during their workout and enabling a greater delivery of oxygen and nutrients to the working muscle. This enhances stamina, endurance and aids muscle repair and growth.

Mode of Action

Cells in the walls of blood vessels produce nitric oxide (NO) from the precursor substrate L-arginine using the enzyme NO synthase (eNOS). NO is a vasodilator which causes blood vessels to relax and helps produce the "pump" experienced by sports people during workouts.

The availability of L-arginine is an essential factor in the production of NO but arginine can also be used by another enzyme called arginase which competes with eNOS for arginine and diverts it away from NO production into other metabolic pathways (the production of ornithine and urea).

Norvaline inhibits the enzyme arginase and hence increases the supply of L-arginine available to be converted into NO by eNOS.

Effectiveness

Norvaline has been demonstrated to effectively inhibit arginase and increase NO production by up to 55% in mouse white blood cells (2) and has shown the ability to vasodilate mouse aortas (a large blood vessel) (3) in *in vitro* experiments.

No experiments have been performed on humans.

Commonly used dosages

Norvaline is usually included as part of a proprietary formulation in commercial sport supplement preparations with the exact quantity of the substance not listed in the ingredients. When the quantity is mentioned, 100mg is the dose most often used.
It is not usually sold as a stand alone supplement.

Due to the absence of human studies it is impossible to comment on a sensible dose of this product.

Safety

No known safety issues.

Interactions

None known.

References

1. Soini J, Falschlehner C, Liedert C, Bernhardt J, Vuoristo J, Neubauer P. Norvaline is accumulated after a down-shift of oxygen in Escherichia coli W3110. Microb Cell Fact. 2008;7:30
2. Chang CI, Liao JC, Kuo L. Arginase modulates nitric oxide production in activated macrophages. Am J Physiol. 1998;274(1 Pt 2):H342-8
3. Ming XF, Barandier C, Viswambharan H, Kwak BR, Mach F *et al*. Thrombin stimulates human endothelial arginase enzymatic activity via RhoA/ROCK pathway: implications for atherosclerotic endothelial dysfunction. Circulation. 2004;110(24):3708-14. Epub 2004 Nov 29

Octopamine

Other names

1-(p-hydroxyphenyl)-2-aminoethanol
Norsympatol
Norsynephrine
Octapamine
Octopaminum
p-hydroxyphenylethanolamine
p-Norsynephrin
α-(Aminomethyl)-4-hydroxybenzenemethanol
α-(aminomethyl)-p-hydroxybenzyl alcohol

Star rating

2

What is it?

A substance found in Seville Oranges, also known as bitter oranges (scientific name: Citrus aurantium) which is structurally similar to norepinephrine (nor-adrenaline). It can be described as a biogenic amine that is the phenol analog of norepinephrine.

It is also produced naturally in the bodies of various animals including humans and was first discovered in octopus salivary glands, hence its name.

The other main active compound found in citrus aurantium is synephrine (see separate entry for synephrine) which is structurally similar to epinephrine (adrenaline). Although both octopamine and synephrine are produced naturally in the human body in very small amounts their exact functions are unknown (1).

Claimed benefits

Fat loss.

Mode of Action

Octopamine is claimed to induce lipolysis (release of fat from fat cells to be used as energy) by stimulating $\beta3$ receptors on fat cells which are presumed to act like $\beta1$ receptors and signal the enzyme hormone sensitive lipase (HSL) to begin breaking down the stored fat.

Humans possess $\beta1$, $\beta2$ and $\beta3$ receptors on fat cells. It is known that activation of β1 and β2 receptors by epinephrine and norepinephrine stimulates HSL to begin lipolysis of stored fat. The discovery that octopamine selectively activates β3 receptors with minimal action on β1and β2 receptors and β3 stimulation causes significant lipolysis in certain animals such as rats, hamsters and dogs led to it being included in sport and weight loss supplements. Its lack of effect on β1and β2 receptors give it the advantage that it should be without the side effects caused by substances which activate these receptors such as increased heart rate etc.

Effectiveness

Unfortunately, research has revealed that there is significant variation between species in the response to activation of β3 receptors. Unlike β1and β2 receptors, β3 receptors play a very minor role in lipolysis in human fat cells and are only activated by very high concentrations of epinephrine and norepinephrine (1) (2) (3).

Octopamine has a much lower affinity for all types of receptors than epinephrine and norepinephrine being between 6000 and 60,000,000 x less potent than norepinephrine in its effect on β receptors (depending on isomer of octopamine used and receptor type) (4) (5).
Given the above it is not surprising then that studies confirm octopamine does not stimulate lipolysis in human cells (6) (7).

Commonly used dosages

Octopamine is usually included in sport supplements in amounts of 100mg – 200mg.

Safety

No known safety issues.

Interactions

None known.

References

1. Fugh-Berman A, Myers A. Citrus aurantium, an ingredient of dietary supplements marketed for weight loss: current status of clinical and basic research. Exp Biol Med (Maywood). 2004;229(8):698-704
2. Galitzky J, Carpéné C, Bousquet-Mélou A, Berlan M, Lafontan M. Differential activation of beta 1-, beta 2- and beta 3-adrenoceptors by catecholamines in white and brown adipocytes. Fundam Clin Pharmacol. 1995;9(4):324-31
3. Lafontan M, Barbe P, Galitzky J, Tavernier G, Langin D *et al.* Adrenergic regulation of adipocyte metabolism. Hum Reprod. 1997;12 Suppl 1:6-20
4. Brown CM, McGrath JC, Midgley JM, Muir AG, O'Brien JW *et al.* Activities of octopamine and synephrine stereoisomers on alpha-adrenoceptors. Br J Pharmacol. 1988;93(2):417-29
5. Jordan R, Midgley JM, Thonoor CM, Williams CM. Beta-adrenergic activities of octopamine and synephrine stereoisomers on guinea-pig atria and trachea. J Pharm Pharmacol. 1987;39(9):752-4
6. Carpéné C, Galitzky J, Fontana E, Atgié C, Lafontan M, Berlan M. Selective activation of beta3-adrenoceptors by octopamine: comparative studies in mammalian fat cells. Naunyn Schmiedebergs Arch Pharmacol. 1999;359(4):310-21

7. Galitzky J, Carpene C, Lafontan M, Berlan M. [Specific stimulation of adipose tissue adrenergic beta 3 receptors by octopamine] [Article in French] C R Acad Sci III. 1993;316(5):519-23

Oleuropein

Other names

2-(3,4-Dihydroxyphenyl)ethyl (2S-(2alpha,3E,4beta))-3-ethylidene-2-(beta-D-glucopyranosyloxy)-3,4-dihydro-5-(methoxycarbonyl)-2H-pyran-4-acetate
Oleuroperin
Oleurpein

Star rating

2

What is it?

A phenolic compound present in olive oil which is present in two forms as oleuropein and aglycone oleuropein. It possesses anti-oxidant properties and is responsible for olive oil's characteristic taste. As with all the beneficial components of olive oil, higher levels are present in extra virgin olive oil since this undergoes virtually no processing.

Claimed benefits

Fat loss.

Mode of Action

Proteins in cells called uncoupling proteins appear able to cause the cell to use more energy for heat production or thermogenesis. Oleuropein seems to able to increase the amount of uncoupling proteins and therefore increase thermogenesis which burns up more calories.

In addition it also stimulates the release of the stimulatory hormones epinephrine (adrenaline) and norepinephrine (noradrenaline) which promote the mobilization of stored fat to be used as energy or used in thermogenesis.

Effectiveness

So far the above mentioned effects have only been observed in studies on rats (1) who had statistically significant less weight gain when fed an oleuropein containing diet than rats fed a control diet.

In this study the thermogenic effect of oleuropein was observed in rat brown adipose tissue. Adult humans have hardly any brown fat but olive oil has also been observed to increase other types of uncoupling proteins in rat white fat tissue and muscle (2) so it is possible that oleuropein can also cause increased thermogenesis in these tissues although this has not been confirmed. There have been no human studies into the effect of oleuropein.

Commonly used dosages

Oleuropin is usually included as part of a proprietary formulation in commercial sport supplement preparations with the exact quantity of the substance not listed in the ingredients.

It is not usually sold as a stand alone supplement.

The lack of human studies make it difficult to estimate a sensible daily intake.

The amount of oleuropein administered to the rats in this study was equivalent to a human consuming 3 – 4g/day which is much higher than it is possible to obtain from consuming olive oil. Oleuropein and oleuropein aglycone are present at approximately 2mg/kg and 19mg/kg in extra virgin olive oil.

Safety

No known safety issues.

Interactions

None known.

References

1. Oi-Kano Y, Kawada T, Watanabe T, Koyama F, Watanabe K, *et al*. Oleuropein, a phenolic compound in extra virgin olive oil, increases uncoupling protein 1 content in brown adipose tissue and enhances noradrenaline and adrenaline secretions in rats. J Nutr Sci Vitaminol (Tokyo). 2008;54(5):363-70
2. Rodríguez VM, Portillo MP, Picó C, Macarulla MT, Palou A. Olive oil feeding up-regulates uncoupling protein genes in rat brown adipose tissue and skeletal muscle. Am J Clin Nutr. 2002;75(2):213-20

Ornithine alpha-ketoglutarate

Other names

L-ornithine alpha-ketoglutarate
OKG
Ornithine ketoglutarate
Ornithine oxoglutarate

Star rating

3

What is it?

A salt composed of two molecules of ornithine and one molecule of α-ketoglutarate. Ornithine is an amino acid which plays a key role in the urea cycle which allows the removal of ammonia from the body. Alpha-ketoglutarate is an intermediate in the Krebs Cycle which is a series of reactions involved in cellular respiration.

Claimed benefits

Anabolic, anti-catabolic, improves body composition, improves recovery from intense exercise.

Mode of Action

Stimulates increased levels of insulin, human growth hormone, IGF-1, nitric oxide and increases glutamine and arginine synthesis.

Effectiveness

There are no studies showing that ornithine alpha-ketoglutarate (OKG) has beneficial effects in healthy sports people or that it has the ability to improve sporting performance.

There are studies showing that OKG has anabolic and anticatabolic actions which speed recovery in burn patients, trauma patients, post surgical patients and in malnourished persons (1) (2) (3) (4) and also increase growth rates in children with retarded growth due to bowel disease (5). These effects seem to be due to the ability of OKG to increase levels of insulin, human growth hormone, IGF-1, nitric oxide and increase glutamine and arginine synthesis.

For example trauma patients receiving 20g/day of OKG mixed into their feed had higher average plasma insulin levels 44.2 µIU/ml compared to 15.7 µIU/ml in patients not receiving OKG and average growth hormone levels of 1.68 ng/ml compared to 0.92 ng/ml in non OKG controls (2).

OKG supplementation has also been tested in healthy individuals. In one study (6) it produced an increase in insulin levels of 24% within 15 minutes when 10g was consumed orally and an increase in plasma arginine levels of 41%. Similar results were obtained in another study on healthy adults also given 10g of OKG (7). Unfortunately growth hormone levels were not measured in these two studies.

In summary OKG has been shown to have an anabolic and anticatabolic action in certain groups of sick people and at least some of the same effects have been demonstrated in healthy adults when OKG is supplemented orally. Further studies are needed to determine what effect long term supplementation with OKG can have in healthy people and whether it can cause significant increases in muscle mass and sporting performance.

Commonly used dosages

There is a wide variation in the amount of OKG contained in commonly available sport supplements from as low as 75mg up to 5 grams.

It is possible to buy OKG as a stand alone supplement, it is most frequently sold in powder form.

Safety

In one of the studies mentioned above (7) 10g of OKG when consumed without food caused a significant hypoglycemia (low blood sugar level) in normal healthy individuals. Consumption of such high doses without food should be avoided.

Interactions

Because OKG increases blood insulin levels there is a theoretical possibility it may increase the effect of diabetes medication. Diabetics should avoid taking OKG.

References

1. Cynober L. Ornithine alpha-ketoglutarate in nutritional support. Nutrition. 1991;7(5):313-22
2. Jeevanandam M, Petersen SR. Substrate fuel kinetics in enterally fed trauma patients supplemented with ornithine alpha ketoglutarate. Clin Nutr. 1999;18(4):209-17
3. Brocker P, Vellas B, Albarede JL, Poynard T. A two-centre, randomized, double-blind trial of ornithine oxoglutarate in 194 elderly, ambulatory, convalescent subjects. Age Ageing. 1994;23(4):303-6

4. Cynober L. Ornithine alpha-ketoglutarate as a potent precursor of arginine and nitric oxide: a new job for an old friend. J Nutr. 2004;134(10 Suppl):2858S-2862S; discussion 2895S

5. Moukarzel AA, Goulet O, Salas JS, Marti-Henneberg C, Buchman AL *et al.* Growth retardation in children receiving long-term total parenteral nutrition: effects of ornithine alpha-ketoglutarate. Am J Clin Nutr. 1994;60(3):408-13

6. Cynober L, Coudray-Lucas C, de Bandt JP, Guéchot J, Aussel C *et al.* Action of ornithine alpha-ketoglutarate, ornithine hydrochloride, and calcium alpha-ketoglutarate on plasma amino acid and hormonal patterns in healthy subjects. J Am Coll Nutr. 1990;9(1):2-12

7. Cynober L, Vaubourdolle M, Dore A, Giboudeau J. Kinetics and metabolic effects of orally administered ornithine alpha-ketoglutarate in healthy subjects fed with a standardized regimen. Am J Clin Nutr. 1984;39(4):514-9

Phenibut

Other names

4-amino-3-phenylbutyric acid
Beta-phenyl-GABA
Beta-phenyl-gamma-aminobutyric acid
Fenibut
Fenigam
Fenigama
Phenigam
Phenigama
Phenigamma
Phenylgamma

Star rating

3

What is it?

Phenibut is a phenyl derivative of the inhibitory neurotransmitter γ-aminobutyric acid or GABA. Phenibut which is considered a neuropsychotropic drug was first synthesized by Perekalin at the Herzen Pedagogic Institute at St. Petersburg in Russia during the 1960's where most of the research into this compound has been published. It is reported to have anxiolytic (calming) and nootropic (cognition enhancing) effects.

Claimed benefits

Sports people use phenibut for its sedative and relaxing properties which promote sleep and aid the body to recover from intense exercise. Some people also use it in the hope of stimulating growth hormone release.

Mode of Action

GABA itself cannot cross the blood brain barrier and therefore has no activity in the brain when consumed orally. The addition of the phenyl ring to GABA allows phenibut to cross the blood brain barrier and be effective when taken orally (1). However the change in structure means that phenibut does not have exactly the same effects as GABA itself.

GABA itself acts on two main receptors GABAA and GABAB. Phenibut is an agonist or activates mainly GABAB receptors but at higher concentrations can also activate GABAA receptors (2). It also appears to act on benzodiazepene (BDZ) receptors but only with long term administration (1).

Other GABAB receptor agonists include the muscle relaxing drug baclofen and the now banned substance GHB. Other GABAA receptor agonists include alcohol, barbiturates and benzodiazepines.

Phenibut can be regarded then as an atypical tranquilizer, sharing some of the characteristics of both benzodiazepines such as diazepam and nootropic drugs such as piracetam. It has mild sedative properties but also seems to enhance learning and memory (1).

Phenibut and Growth Hormone: Other GABA receptor agonists such as baclofen and GHB can increase levels of growth hormone in healthy adults (3) (4). It is entirely possible that phenibut also has this effect but no studies have yet been done to confirm this. It is known that phenibut increases dopamine levels in rat brains which is a known mechanism of GH release in humans (1).

Effectiveness

Despite being reportedly used quite frequently in Russia in the treatment of neurological and psychiatric disorders few human studies on phenibut have been reported. In the few studies which have been done, mainly in Russia, phenibut has been reported to alleviate anxiety, be a useful tranquilizer and to enhance intellectual function in geriatric patients. In children it has been used successfully in the treatment of hyperactivity, insomnia and stuttering (1).

In animal studies phenibut has been demonstrated to have a diazepam-like tranquilizing effect, enhances learning, enhances the effect of anesthetic and anti-seizure medication and alleviates withdrawal symptoms from alcohol and morphine (1).

No specific studies exist regarding the ability of phenibut to promote recovery from exercise.

Commonly used dosages

Phenibut is most often sold as a stand alone product either as a free powder or in capsules ranging from 250mg to 500mg and with a recommended dose of up to 1500mg if taken to improve sleep. It can also sometimes be found as a component of "GH releasing" formulas.

The Russian studies reported that tolerance to the effects of phenibut appear quite rapidly and that after two weeks the dose had to be increased by up to one third in some patients (1).

Safety

In human studies in Russia doses of 1500mg/day appear to

have been safe in geriatric patients for periods of up to two weeks and no toxic effects have been reported. Phenibut has a plasma half life of 5.3 hours and is mainly excreted in the urine (1).

Interactions

Phenibut may increase the effect of anesthetics, anti seizure medications, alcohol, opioid pain killers, sleeping pills and benzodiazepines such as diazepam. It should be avoided by anyone taking any of these kinds of medication.

References

1. Lapin I. Phenibut (beta-phenyl-GABA): a tranquilizer and nootropic drug. CNS Drug Rev. 2001;7(4):471-81
2. Shulgina GI. On neurotransmitter mechanisms of reinforcement and internal inhibition. Pavlov J Biol Sci. 1986;21(4):129-40
3. Volpi R, Chiodera P, Caffarra P, Scaglioni A, Malvezzi L *et al.* Muscarinic cholinergic mediation of the GH response to gamma-hydroxybutyric acid: neuroendocrine evidence in normal and parkinsonian subjects. Psychoneuroendocrinology. 2000;25(2):179-85
4. Volpi R, Chiodera P, Caffarra P, Scaglioni A, Saccani A, Coiro V. Different control mechanisms of growth hormone (GH) secretion between gamma-amino- and gamma-hydroxy-butyric acid: neuroendocrine evidence in Parkinson's disease. Psychoneuroendocrinology. 1997;22(7):531-8

Raspberry Ketones

Other names

4-(4-hydroxyphenyl) butan-2-one
Frambinone
Oxyphenylon
p-hydroxybutanone
Rasketone
Rheosmin

Star rating

2

What is it?

A phenolic compound found in raspberries (Rubus idaeus) which is responsible for their unique aroma and which has a structure similar to the structures of the anti-obesity compounds capsaicin and synephrine (1). It is widely used as a food flavouring in the food industry. Low amounts are produced naturally by the plants, only between 1 to 17 μg/100g FW which makes the natural product an expensive compound. However the ketones can also be produced synthetically and more cheaply by chemical processes and also from cultures of certain strains of bacteria (2).

Claimed benefits

Fat loss.

Mode of Action

Raspberry ketones increase norepinephrine (noradrenaline) induced lipolysis in white adipocytes (1) and may also increase levels of the hormone adiponectin which appears to play a role in the regulation of fatty acid breakdown. Obese people have lower levels of adiponectin (3).

Effectiveness

The anti-obesity of effects of raspberry ketones have only been tested in one study on mice. Mice fed a high fat diet including 0.5, 1, or 2% of raspberry ketones for 10 weeks did not gain weight compared to mice fed the same high fat diet without the raspberry ketones. In addition mice who had gained weight on a high fat diet then lost weight when raspberry ketones were added to their diet for 5 weeks (1).

Commonly used dosages

Raspberry ketones are usually included as part of a proprietary formulation in commercial sport supplement preparations with the exact quantity of the substance not listed in the ingredients.

When the exact amount is given quantities from 125mg to 200mg can be seen.

There are few stand-alone raspberry ketone products on the market.

Safety

No known safety issues.

Interactions

None known.

References

1. Morimoto C, Satoh Y, Hara M, Inoue S, Tsujita T, Okuda H. Anti-obese action of raspberry ketone. Life Sci. 2005;77(2):194-204. Epub 2005 Feb 25
2. MetaCyc Pathway: raspberry ketone biosynthesis [online] at http://biocyc.org/META/new-image?type=PATHWAY&object=PWY-5393
3. Park KS. Raspberry ketone increases both lipolysis and fatty acid oxidation in 3T3-L1 adipocytes. Planta Med. 2010;76(15):1654-8. Epub 2010 Apr 27

Resveratrol

Other names

trans - resveratrol
(E)-5-(p-hydroxystyryl)resorcinol
3,5,4'-trihydroxystilbene
3,4',5-stilbenetriol
5-[(1E)-2-(4-hydroxyphenyl)ethenyl]-1,3-benzenediol

Star rating

2

What is it?

A polyphenolic phytoalexin (plant anti-microbial substance) which is structurally very similar to the synthetic estrogen diethylstilbestrol. It is present in a variety of food sources most notably grapes (Vitis vinifera) and red wine and much of the research into resveratrol arose due to epidemiological studies showing an inverse relationship between moderate red wine consumption and cardiovascular disease risk, the so called "French paradox". The phenomena whereby certain segments of the French population are less susceptible to heart diseases despite their high fat diet, (1).

Resveratrol occurs naturally in two forms as isomers, trans-(E) and cis- (Z) resveratrol. The trans form demonstrates much greater binding capacity for the estrogen receptor ER and is therefore mainly responsible for the beneficial effects of resveratrol (2) (3).

In most wines about two thirds of the resveratrol content is the trans form and one third the cis form. The total resveratrol content of wine depends on the type of grape, the region of cultivation and the type of yeast used in its fermentation. Red wines contain the highest amounts with quantities ranging from approximately 1 to 6 mg/L. In particular Merlot and Pinot Noir wines contain the highest amounts and French and Spanish red wines in general contain high quantities (4). White wines contain less than 5% of the resveratrol content of red wines (1).

Other foods containing high levels of resveratrol include red grape juice (~0.50 mg/L), cranberry juice (~0.2 mg/L), grapes (0.16–3.54 µg/g) and peanuts (0.02–1.92 µg/g). The traditional Chinese and Japanese herb *Polygonum cuspidatum* used as a remedy for various ailments including fungal infections and cardiovascular illness also contains high amounts (5).

Most of the research conducted on resveratrol has focused on its promising anti-atherosclerosis, cholesterol improving and anti-cancer effects. However I will concentrate my discussion on its use in sport supplements which centers around its anti-estrogenic effects.

Claimed benefits

Acts as an anti-estrogen which helps to limit fat gain and indirectly increases testosterone production via reduced estrogenic negative feedback to the hypothalamus and pituitary gland.

Mode of Action

Resveratrol has been observed to have both estrogenic and anti-estrogenic effects, mainly in *in vitro* tests on human breast cancer cells (6) (7) (8) (9). This has led some to propose that it may function as a selective estrogen receptor modulator (SERM) like the prescription breast cancer drug tamoxifen.

SERM's such as tamoxifen act like estrogen in some tissues e.g. blood vessels and bone improving cardiovascular health and bone density but block the action of estrogen in other tissues such as the breast which helps prevent the growth of breast tumors.

SERM's also act to block the effect of estrogen in the hypothalamus and pituitary gland. By reducing the negative feedback signals from estrogen the pituitary gland is stimulated to increase output of luteinizing hormone LH and follicle stimulating hormone FSH which in turn increase production of the sex hormones, estrogen in women and testosterone in men. For this reason tamoxifen is also used in the treatment of male and female infertility.

Resveratrol has also been found to act as an aromatase inhibitor in *in vitro* cell studies. It can reduce estrogen levels by inhibiting the action of the enzyme aromatase which converts androgens into estrogen (10).

Effectiveness

The theory that resveratrol can increase testosterone production has been demonstrated in one animal study. Rats fed 20mg/kg body weight per day of resveratrol for 90 days had nearly a 100% increase in their LH and FSH levels and nearly a 200% increase in their testosterone levels. Sperm counts also increased and the rats had no adverse effects from the resveratrol (11).

However there are several good reasons to believe that this effect may not be applicable to humans.

First of all estrogen receptor physiology is complex and not completely understood. There are significant differences in estrogen receptor response between species and different tissues and cells. Human responses may not be equivalent to rats (12).

Second is the issue of dosing. The rats in this study were given a dose of 20mg/kg an amount equivalent to 1400mg for a 70kg man. This is 1000 times more than the amount of resveratrol that could obtained from drinking 250ml of red wine and many times the recommended dose of resveratrol supplements which usually come in capsules of 100mg. Such high doses could have adverse health consequences as we will discuss below.

It should be noted that very low blood concentrations of resveratrol such as those likely to be obtained from red wine are in the range capable of exerting protective effects on the cardiovascular system by increasing levels of nitric oxide which acts as an anti-oxidant and vasorelaxant and by reducing platelet aggregation.

However most of the other effects observed in the tests

discussed above such as anti-estrogenic effects, aromatase inhibition, anti-cancer effects etc. are only observed at much higher concentrations (5) which would require an oral ingestion of at least 5 grams of resveratrol in humans (13).

Commonly used dosages

Resveratrol is included in a variety of sport supplements in amounts from under 100mg up to 300mg.

It is also sold as a stand alone supplement, usually in capsules of 100mg with recommended daily intake of two capsules.

Safety

The consumption of a single dose of 5 grams of resveratrol was found to be safe in humans although the effects of long term consumption at this level are unknown (13).

There is some evidence that while resveratrol has beneficial effects at low doses, at high doses it may begin to have adverse effects. At low doses it functions as an anti-oxidant but at high doses may function as a pro-oxidant. At low concentrations it protects blood vessels by increasing nitric oxide in endothelial cells but at high concentrations it can cause endothelial cell apoptosis (cell death). Hypercholesterolemic rabbits given high doses of resveratrol develop atherosclerosis faster than rabbits not given resveratrol.

In cancer studies high concentrations of resveratrol caused death of cancer cells but also reduced growth and caused the death of some normal cells (5).

While these risks may be worthwhile in the treatment of

conditions such as cancer they would be hard to justify for healthy individuals while the benefits of high dose resveratrol supplementation remain so uncertain.

Interactions

Resveratrol inhibits platelet aggregation which increases the amount of time it takes for the blood to clot (14). There is a theoretical possibility it could increase the effect of other anti-platelet drugs such as aspirin, ibuprofen, diclofenac etc. or of anti-coagulant drugs such as heparin and warfarin (coumarin) leading to increased bruising or bleeding. Anyone taking these kinds of medicines should avoid taking resveratrol.

References

1. Pervaiz S. Resveratrol: from grapevines to mammalian biology. FASEB J. 2003;17(14):1975-85
2. Abou-Zeid LA, El-Mowafy AM. Differential recognition of resveratrol isomers by the human estrogen receptor-alpha: molecular dynamics evidence for stereoselective ligand binding. Chirality. 2004;16(3):190-5
3. Basly JP, Marre-Fournier F, Le Bail JC, Habrioux G, Chulia AJ. Estrogenic/antiestrogenic and scavenging properties of (E)- and (Z)-resveratrol. Life Sci. 2000;66(9):769-77
4. Gu X, Creasy L, Kester A, Zeece M. Capillary electrophoretic determination of resveratrol in wines. J Agric Food Chem. 1999;47(8):3223-7
5. Mukherjee S, Dudley JI, Das DK. Dose-dependency of resveratrol in providing health benefits. Dose Response. 2010;8(4):478-500
6. Bowers JL, Tyulmenkov VV, Jernigan SC, Klinge CM. Resveratrol acts as a mixed agonist/antagonist for

estrogen receptors alpha and beta. Endocrinology. 2000;141(10):3657-67

7. Basly JP, Marre-Fournier F, Le Bail JC, Habrioux G, Chulia AJ. Estrogenic/antiestrogenic and scavenging properties of (E)- and (Z)-resveratrol. Life Sci. 2000 Jan 21;66(9):769-77

8. Gehm BD, McAndrews JM, Chien PY, Jameson JL. Resveratrol, a polyphenolic compound found in grapes and wine, is an agonist for the estrogen receptor. Proc Natl Acad Sci U S A. 1997 Dec;94(25):14138-43

9. Lu R, Serrero G. Resveratrol, a natural product derived from grape, exhibits antiestrogenic activity and inhibits the growth of human breast cancer cells. J Cell Physiol. 1999;179(3):297-304

10. Wang Y, Lee KW, Chan FL, Chen S, Leung LK. The red wine polyphenol resveratrol displays bilevel inhibition on aromatase in breast cancer cells. Toxicol Sci. 2006;92(1):71-7. Epub 2006 Apr 11

11. Juan ME, González-Pons E, Munuera T, Ballester J, Rodríguez-Gil JE, Planas JM. trans-Resveratrol, a natural antioxidant from grapes, increases sperm output in healthy rats. J Nutr. 2005;135(4):757-60

12. Kuiper GG, Shughrue PJ, Merchenthaler I, Gustafsson JA. The estrogen receptor beta subtype: a novel mediator of estrogen action in neuroendocrine systems. Front Neuroendocrinol. 1998;19(4):253-86

13. Boocock DJ, Faust GE, Patel KR, Schinas AM, Brown VA *et al*. Phase I dose escalation pharmacokinetic study in healthy volunteers of resveratrol, a potential cancer chemopreventive agent. Cancer Epidemiol Biomarkers Prev. 2007;16(6):1246-52

14. Pace-Asciak CR, Rounova O, Hahn SE, Diamandis EP, Goldberg DM. Wines and grape juices as modulators of platelet aggregation in healthy human subjects. Clin Chim Acta. 1996 Mar;246(1-2):163-82

Rhodiola rosea

Other names

Arctic root
Golden root
Orpin rose
Rhodiole Rougeatre
Rosenroot
Roseroot
Sedum rhodiola
Sedum rosea

Star rating

4

What is it?

A plant of the family Crassulaceae which grows in mountain
rock crevices in the arctic regions of Europe, Asia and North
America. It has a long history of use in traditional medicine
particularly in Northern Europe as far back as the Vikings. It
has been used as a treatment for headaches, kidney stones,
skin conditions, a general stimulant and tonic.

Most of the modern interest in Rhodiola has come from
Russia where much research has been carried out since the
1960's, whereas "western" researchers only began to become
interested in Rhodiola in the mid 1980's. The
Pharmacological Committee of the Ministry of Health in the
USSR recommended the use of Rhodiola as a stimulant in
1969 (1).

Claimed benefits

Increases energy, stamina and functions as an adaptogen helping the organism to withstand physical and mental stress. It is often included in post work-out formulas as it is believed to aid in recovery from exercise.

Mode of Action

Rhodiola contains a large number of constituent compounds including flavonoids, phenylethanoids, phenylpropanoids, piceins, sterols, tannins and volatile oils (2). Many of these have pharmacological actions including anti-depressive, anti-fatigue, liver protective, nootropic, anti-oxidant, cardio-protective and anti-inflammatory effects however the compound which has most activity and is believed to be responsible for most of the adaptogenic effects of Rhodiola is salidroside (also called (rhodioloside or p-hydroxyphenylethyl-O-β-d-glucopyranoside). Various other salidroside-like compounds may also be important such as rhodiolin, rosin, rosavin, rosarin, and rosiridin.

Rhodiola exerts its adaptogenic effects by having a normalizing effect on the hormonal and chemical changes caused in the body by stress.

Mental and physical stress, including stress caused by moderate and intense exercise, (but not low intensity exercise) causes increased levels of the hormone cortisol (3) (4). While cortisol plays an important role in helping the body to cope with stress, mainly via its anti-inflammatory effects it also has undesirable effects which sports people in particular may be interested in minimizing or reducing as quickly as possible after exercise.

Cortisol causes reduced transport of amino acids into

muscles and increases transport of amino acids out of muscles resulting in decreased protein synthesis and increased protein catabolism. In addition cortisol suppresses RNA formation which further reduces protein synthesis particularly in muscle. In addition cortisol causes many cells particularly muscles to become insulin resistant (5).

Finally, while in the short term cortisol causes fatty acids to be mobilized from fat tissue to be used for energy, chronically high levels of cortisol can cause increased obesity and is associated particularly with abdominal obesity and increased intra-abdominal or visceral fat (6).

Rhodiola reduces cortisol levels (1) (7) and increases the production of other stress defence mechanism proteins such as Hsp 70 which reduces the stress-induced increase in nitric oxide, and the associated decrease in ATP production which results in increased performance and endurance (8).

Effectiveness

A systematic review (1) of hundreds of Rhodiola studies including 30 human trials of which three were randomized controlled trials and eleven placebo controlled trials confirmed the effect of Rhodiola as an adaptogen.

Significant beneficial specific effects of reducing stress induced fatigue and improving attention and mental performance were found. The inhibitory effect of Rhodiola on cortisol levels was also confirmed which the review states "is in line with other studies demonstrating that optimal corticosteroid levels are a requirement for efficient cognitive function".

These effects are seen both after chronic long term

supplementation and acute one off administration of Rhodiola.

Results of clinical trials examining the physical performance enhancing effects of Rhodiola have been conflicting. Two studies have reported improvements. One showed that four weeks supplementation of Rhodiola in 14 trained male athletes reduced plasma free fatty acid levels, blood lactate and markers of skeletal muscle damage after exhaustive exercise (9). Another double blind randomized controlled trial with 24 participants showed that a one off dose of 200mg Rhodiola extract improved endurance exercise capacity when taken one hour beforehand. Confusingly however taking the same dose daily for 4 weeks beforehand did not improve endurance (10). In a further study carried out with the Polish national rowing team, rowers taking 100mg twice daily for four weeks showed increased antioxidant levels in their blood but no reduction in oxidative damage induced by exhaustive exercise (11).

Two further studies failed to show any effect of Rhodiola supplementation on perceived fatigue, time to exhaustion or muscle tissue oxygen saturation in exercising individuals (12) (13).

While these results show that Rhodiola supplementation has uncertain benefit for endurance athletes, all the studies performed were of insufficient duration to measure any long term anabolic effect which could be expected from lower cortisol levels and the increased protein synthesis this would promote. Further studies are needed to assess this.

Commonly used dosages

Rhodiola rosea is often included as part of a proprietary formulation in commercial sport supplement preparations with the exact quantity of the substance not listed in the ingredients.

When an amount is listed in the ingredients a wide variety of doses can be seen from as low as 10mg up to 400mg.

Extracts of Rhodiola rosea are usually standardized to contain a certain percentage of both salidroside and rosavin (typically 3% rosavin and 1% salidroside). This is due to the fact that salidroside can be found in various species of Rhodiola while rosavin is found only in Rhodiola rosea. Extracts of Rhodiola rosea are therefore standardized by its unique rosavin content (14).

The therapeutic dose of Rhodiola will depend on the degree of standardization as measured by the rosavin content. For a 1% rosavin content a regular daily dose of 360mg to 600mg is suggested. For a 3.6% rosavin content the dose would be 100mg to 170mg.

For a one off acute dose taken just before a stressful situation the above amounts should be multiplied by three (14).

It is also important to note that the effect of Rhodiola does not follow a linear dose-effect response. In other words taking more does not mean more results. Rhodiola is ineffective in low doses, effective at moderate doses and ineffective again at high doses (1).

The Russian approach to adaptogen administration has generally been to take the adaptogen in repeated short cycles (14).

Safety

No known safety issues. There have been reports of some

individuals experiencing irritability and insomnia at high doses over 1500mg per day (14).

Interactions

None known.

References

1. Panossian A, Wikman G, Sarris J. Rosenroot (Rhodiola rosea): traditional use, chemical composition, pharmacology and clinical efficacy. Phytomedicine. 2010;17(7):481-93. Epub 2010 Apr 7
2. Barnes J, Anderson LA, Phillipson JD. Herbal Medicines. 3rd ed. London: Pharmaceutical Press; 2007
3. Hill EE, Zack E, Battaglini C, Viru M, Viru A, Hackney AC. Exercise and circulating cortisol levels: the intensity threshold effect. J Endocrinol Invest. 2008;31(7):587-91
4. Hough JP, Papacosta E, Wraith E, Gleeson M. Plasma and salivary steroid hormone responses of men to high-intensity cycling and resistance exercise. J Strength Cond Res. 2011;25(1):23-31
5. Guyton AC, Hall JE. Textbook of Medical Physiology 11th Ed. Philadelphia: Elsevier Saunders; 2006
6. Purnell JQ, Kahn SE, Samuels MH, Brandon D, Loriaux DL, Brunzell JD. Enhanced cortisol production rates, free cortisol, and 11beta-HSD-1 expression correlate with visceral fat and insulin resistance in men: effect of weight loss. Am J Physiol Endocrinol Metab. 2009;296(2):E351-7. Epub 2008 Dec 2
7. Olsson EM, von Schéele B, Panossian AG. A randomised, double-blind, placebo-controlled, parallel-group study of the standardised extract shr-5 of the roots of Rhodiola rosea in the treatment of subjects with stress-related fatigue. Planta Med. 2009;75(2):105-12. Epub 2008 Nov 18

8. Panossian A, Wikman G. Evidence-based efficacy of adaptogens in fatigue, and molecular mechanisms related to their stress-protective activity. Curr Clin Pharmacol. 2009;4(3):198-219. Epub 2009 Sep 1

9. Parisi A, Tranchita E, Duranti G, Ciminelli E, Quaranta F *et al.* Effects of chronic Rhodiola Rosea supplementation on sport performance and antioxidant capacity in trained male: preliminary results. J Sports Med Phys Fitness. 2010;50(1):57-63

10. De Bock K, Eijnde BO, Ramaekers M, Hespel P. Acute Rhodiola rosea intake can improve endurance exercise performance. Int J Sport Nutr Exerc Metab. 2004;14(3):298-307

11. Skarpanska-Stejnborn A, Pilaczynska-Szczesniak L, Basta P, Deskur-Smielecka E. The influence of supplementation with Rhodiola rosea L. extract on selected redox parameters in professional rowers. Int J Sport Nutr Exerc Metab. 2009;19(2):186-99

12. Colson SN, Wyatt FB, Johnston DL, Autrey LD, FitzGerald YL, Earnest CP. Cordyceps sinensis- and Rhodiola rosea-based supplementation in male cyclists and its effect on muscle tissue oxygen saturation. J Strength Cond Res. 2005;19(2):358-63

13. Walker TB, Altobelli SA, Caprihan A, Robergs RA. Failure of Rhodiola rosea to alter skeletal muscle phosphate kinetics in trained men. Metabolism. 2007;56(8):1111-7

14. Kelly GS. Rhodiola rosea: a possible plant adaptogen. Altern Med Rev. 2001;6(3):293-302

Sesamin / Episesamin

Other names

Sesame lignan
Sesame seed
Sesamum indicum

Star rating

2

What is it?

Oil extracted from the seeds of the flowering plant Sesame in the genus Sesamum found in many tropical regions of the world. It is grown primarily for its seeds which are used in cooking.

In sport and health supplements the oil extracted from the seeds is used.

Claimed benefits

Fat loss and reduced fat storage.

Mode of Action

Sesame seeds contain compounds called lignans. The main lignans found are sesamin, sesamolin and sesaminol. Sesaminol is not extractable in oil and during the refining process sesamolin degrades leaving mainly sesamin. However during the refining process sesamin is also affected and is epimerized to episesamin hence commercially available sesame oil contains sesamin and episesamin in a ratio of 1:1 (1).

Both sesamin and episesamin have been found in various studies on rats to increase the rate at which rat liver cells oxidize fat (use it for energy) and reduce the rate at which fat is stored (1) (2) (3) (4) (5).

Cells contain organelles called peroxisomes and mitochondria which are both involved in the metabolism of fats. Sesamin and episesamin both increase liver mitochondrial and peroxisomal fatty acid oxidation and also increase the activity and gene expression of various fatty acid oxidation enzymes.

It was also observed that these lignans reduced the gene expression of various proteins involved in hepatic lipogenesis (fat storage), cholesterol formation and glucose metabolism.

Of the two lignans episesamin was found to have a more powerful effect than sesamin multiplying mitochondrial and peroxisomal activity by 2.3 and 5.1 fold compared to 1.7 and 1.6 for sesamin. Episesamin also increased the activity of fatty acid oxidation enzymes up to 14 fold compared to 2.8 fold for sesamin (2).

Effectiveness

Although the ability of sesame lignans to increase fat oxidation in rat liver cells is impressive it is unknown whether this would actually translate into measurable fat loss in either rats or humans since this does not appear to have been tested at the current time.

Commonly used dosages

Sesame is often included as part of a proprietary formulation in commercial sport supplement preparations with the exact quantity of the substance not listed in the ingredients. When listed, amounts of 1000mg are common. Some supplements specifically state that the sesame oil included has been standardized to contain a standard amount of sesamin, typically 50% however many do not.

Thus far supplements standardized to contain higher amounts of the more powerful episesamin have not been seen on the market.

Sesamin can also be found as a stand alone supplement in capsules containing 500mg to 1000mg with recommended intakes of 3 capsules daily.

Safety

No known safety issues.

Interactions

None known.

References

1. Ide T, Nakashima Y, Iida H, Yasumoto S, Katsuta M. Lipid metabolism and nutrigenomics - impact of sesame lignans on gene expression profiles and fatty acid oxidation in rat liver. Forum Nutr. 2009;61:10-24. Epub 2009 Apr 7
2. Kushiro M, Masaoka T, Hageshita S, Takahashi Y, Ide T, Sugano M. Comparative effect of sesamin and episesamin on the activity and gene expression of enzymes in fatty acid oxidation and synthesis in rat liver. J Nutr Biochem. 2002;13(5):289-295
3. Sirato-Yasumoto S, Katsuta M, Okuyama Y, Takahashi Y, Ide T. Effect of sesame seeds rich in sesamin and

sesamolin on fatty acid oxidation in rat liver. J Agric
Food Chem. 2001;49(5):2647-51

4. Ashakumary L, Rouyer I, Takahashi Y, Ide T, Fukuda N
et al. Sesamin, a sesame lignan, is a potent inducer of
hepatic fatty acid oxidation in the rat. Metabolism.
1999;48(10):1303-13

5. Ide T, Lim JS, Odbayar TO, Nakashima Y. Comparative
study of sesame lignans (sesamin, episesamin and
sesamolin) affecting gene expression profile and fatty
acid oxidation in rat liver. J Nutr Sci Vitaminol (Tokyo).
2009;55(1):31-43

Sodium D - Aspartate

Other names

(2R)-2-aminobutanedioic acid
(R)-Aspartic acid
Aspartic acid D-form
Aspartic acid, D-
DADAVIT ®
D-Aspartate
D-Aspartic acid

Star rating

3

What is it?

All amino acids exist as stereoisomers in L and D forms (two
forms which differ only in the three-dimensional orientation
of their atoms). D-aspartate is a naturally occurring amino
acid first discovered in the nervous system of molluscs. It has

since also been found in the nervous and endocrine systems of various other animals including humans where it is believed to play a role in the biosynthesis and release of sex hormones (1).

In mammals D-aspartate is found concentrated in the brain, pineal gland, pituitary gland and testes and mammalian cells appear able to synthesize, release, take up, and degrade the amino acid (2).

Claimed benefits

Increases testosterone levels.

Mode of Action

D-aspartate appears able to increase testosterone in two ways. Firstly it stimulates the production of luteinizing hormone (LH) in the pituitary gland. Luteinizing hormone as we know stimulates the Leydig cells in the testes to produce more testosterone.

Secondly D-aspartate increases the amount of testosterone the testes are able to produce in response to LH. Testosterone is produced in the Leydig cells from cholesterol which has to be transported into the cell by a transport protein called Steroidogenic Acute Regulatory protein (StAR). The amount of cholesterol which can be transported into the cell is the rate limiting step in testosterone synthesis. D-aspartate enters the Leydig cells via a L-Glu transporter and causes the cell nucleus to produce more StAR protein (2) (3) (4).

Effectiveness

Two studies have confirmed the ability of D-aspartate to

increase LH and testosterone levels in rats.

In the first, D-aspartate accumulated in the pituitary and testes to 12 and 4 times basal levels when given to rats and this caused a 60% increase in LH levels and a 190% increase in testosterone levels (5).

In the second, rats given a D-aspartate solution to drink for 12 days showed a 51% increase in LH levels compared to controls and a 105% increase in testosterone levels. Three days after suspension of treatment the rats still showed a statistically significant 20% increase in testosterone levels, probably due to the accumulation of D-aspartate in the testes (1).

In the same study 23 human males at an IVF (in vitro fertilization) Unit took a commercially available formulation of 3.12g sodium D-aspartate (DADAVIT ®) also containing Vitamin B6, Folic Acid and Vitamin B12 and marketed as a supplement to increase the quality of human seminal fluid. A placebo group of 20 men were given an identical formulation containing the same vitamins but no D-aspartate.

After 6 days LH levels were virtually unchanged but after 12 days 20 of the participants had a statistically significant increase in LH levels of 33%. There was no change in the placebo group. Testosterone levels followed a similar pattern with a small but non significant rise after 6 days but by day 12 there was a rise of 42%. Three days after suspension of treatment testosterone levels were still elevated by 22%.

Commonly used dosages

D-aspartate is usually sold as a stand alone supplement in the form of a powder with a recommended dose of 3g.

DADAVIT ® the product used in the human study cited above is produced by the Italian company Pharmaguida S.r.l. and can be purchased as a non prescription supplement from Italian pharmacies and web sites. It comes in boxes of 15 vials of 10ml of liquid containing 3.12g sodium D–aspartate (5).

Safety

No known safety issues.

Interactions

None known.

References

1. Topo E, Soricelli A, D'Aniello A, Ronsini S, D'Aniello G. The role and molecular mechanism of D-aspartic acid in the release and synthesis of LH and testosterone in humans and rats. Reprod Biol Endocrinol. 2009;7:120
2. Furuchi T, Homma H. Free D-aspartate in mammals. Biol Pharm Bull. 2005;28(9):1566-70
3. Nagata Y, Homma H, Matsumoto M, Imai K. Stimulation of steroidogenic acute regulatory protein (StAR) gene expression by D-aspartate in rat Leydig cells. FEBS Lett. 1999;454(3):317-20
4. Nagata Y, Homma H, Lee JA, Imai K. D-Aspartate stimulation of testosterone synthesis in rat Leydig cells. FEBS Lett. 1999;444(2-3):160-4
5. Pharmaguida, DADAVIT, [online] at http://www.pharmaguida.com/eng/dadavit.asp

Synephrine

Other names

1-(4-hydroxyphenyl)-2-methylaminoethanol
4-Hydroxy-α-[(methylamino)methyl]benzenemethanol
methylaminomethyl 4-hydroxyphenyl carbinol
Oxedrine
p-hydroxy-α-[(methylamino)methyl]benzyl alcohol
p-methylaminoethanolphenol
p-Synephrine
Synephrin
β-methylamino-α-(4-hydroxyphenyl)ethyl alcohol

Star rating

3

What is it?

A substance found in Seville Oranges, also known as bitter oranges (scientific name: Citrus aurantium) which is structurally similar to epinephrine (adrenaline).

It is also produced naturally in the bodies of various animals including humans and can be classified as an alpha adrenergic agonist having activity mainly at the α1 receptor but also weakly at the α2 receptor. It also has activity at the β3 receptor and weak activity at the β1 receptor with virtually no action at β2 (1) (2) (3).

The other main active compound found in citrus aurantium is octopamine (see separate entry for octopamine) which is structurally similar to norepinephrine (noradrenaline). Although both octopamine and synephrine are produced naturally in the human body in very small amounts their exact functions are unknown (1).

Claimed benefits

Fat loss and appetite suppression.

Mode of Action

Synephrine's action can be considered according to the response stimulated by each receptor type:

Stimulation of $\alpha 1$ receptors causes vasoconstriction, which leads to an increase in blood pressure. Stimulation of $\alpha 2$ receptors causes vasodilation and also inhibits lipolysis (inhibits the break down of stored fats to be used for energy) (4). As we have seen synephrine activates $\alpha 2$ receptors only weakly.

Stimulation of $\beta 1$ receptors initiates lipolysis by signalling the enzyme hormone sensitive lipase (HSR) to begin breaking down stored fat to be used for energy. It also causes an increased heart rate (4).

Stimulation of $\beta 3$ receptors causes thermogenesis (increased heat production) in brown fat, however adults have virtually no brown fat, so this effect can be considered negligible. It is claimed that $\beta 3$ receptors also cause lipolysis, however while this is true in certain animals such as rats, hamsters and dogs $\beta 3$ receptors play a very minor role in lipolysis in human fat cells and are only activated by very high concentrations of epinephrine and norepinephrine (1) (5) (6).

Synephrine binds to β receptors between 100 and 400 million times less strongly than norepinephrine (depending which receptor and isomer of synephrine is used), so it is extremely unlikely that synephrine is responsible for any lipolytic action via this receptor (3).

Effectiveness

Studies show that synephrine is capable of increasing blood pressure and heart rate for up to five hours (7) (8) and transiently increasing resting metabolic rate although no appetite suppressing effect was observed (9).

This indicates it is at least capable of a mild stimulatory effect as would be predicted from its receptor interaction.

Whether this translates into any appreciable fat loss is much less certain. Several reviews of all the available trials testing synephrine for fat loss have been reported and most have concluded that at the present time there is insufficient evidence to recommend its use (1) (10) (11) (12).

Commonly used dosages

Both synephrine and citrus aurantium are usually included as part of a proprietary formulation in commercial sport supplement preparations with the exact quantity of the substance not listed in the ingredients.

When the amount is listed amounts from 5mg to 30mg can be seen.

I have seen only one stand alone synephrine product available which is Syn-30 produced by Serious Nutrition Solutions and which contains 30mg of pure synephrine HCl.

Safety

Although either synephrine itself or citrus aurantium has been used safely for short periods of time in the various studies mentioned above there have been a few reports of adverse events occurring in some individuals associated with its use.

In most cases the individuals concerned were taking weight loss products containing various ingredients including synephrine so it is hard to say for certain to what extent the other ingredients are to blame if at all. However in some cases at least it is likely that the synephrine content was responsible. These adverse events include myocardial infarction (heart attack) (13), angina (14), cardiac arrhythmia (15), tachycardia (16) and stroke (17).

Anyone with any history of stroke, heart problems or high blood pressure should not take synephrine.

Interactions

Due to its stimulatory effects synephrine may increase the effect of other stimulatory compounds such as caffeine and in particular may cause increased blood pressure if taken with cold and flu medications which contain pseudoephedrine due to its similar chemical structure. For similar reasons synephrine may also interfere with the action of anti-hypertension medication. Anyone taking blood pressure medication or medication containing pseudoephedrine should not take synephrine.

Synephrine may also dangerously increase blood pressure if taken with a class of anti-depressant medications called MAOI's (monoamine oxidase inhibitors). If you take a MAOI anti-depressant you should not take synephrine (18).

Citrus aurantium extract has been found to have the same effect on the metabolism of some drugs as grapefruit, probably due to the compound bergapten which is contained in both. Bergapten down-regulates the cytochrome P450 enzyme CYP3A4 which breaks down many drugs and so both citrus aurantium and grapefruit could dangerously increase drug levels in the blood (19) (20).

Therefore it would be cautious to avoid taking citrus aurantium with any drug known to be affected by grapefruit, of which there are many. These include anti-arrhythmics, anti-malarials, anxiolytics, calcium channel blockers, ciclosporin, lipid regulating drugs, sildenafil, tadalafil, vardenafil and tacrolimus. Please consult your doctor if in any doubt. This does not apply to pure synephrine, only supplements containing the whole citrus aurantium extract.

References

1. Fugh-Berman A, Myers A. Citrus aurantium, an ingredient of dietary supplements marketed for weight loss: current status of clinical and basic research. Exp Biol Med (Maywood). 2004;229(8):698-704
2. Brown CM, McGrath JC, Midgley JM, Muir AG, O'Brien JW *et al.* Activities of octopamine and synephrine stereoisomers on alpha-adrenoceptors. Br J Pharmacol. 1988;93(2):417-29
3. Jordan R, Midgley JM, Thonoor CM, Williams CM. Beta-adrenergic activities of octopamine and synephrine stereoisomers on guinea-pig atria and trachea. J Pharm Pharmacol. 1987;39(9):752-4
4. Tortora GJ, Derrickson B. Principles of Anatomy and Physiology 11th Ed. New Jersey: John Wiley & Sons Inc; 2006

5. Galitzky J, Carpéné C, Bousquet-Mélou A, Berlan M, Lafontan M. Differential activation of beta 1-, beta 2- and beta 3-adrenoceptors by catecholamines in white and brown adipocytes. Fundam Clin Pharmacol. 1995;9(4):324-31

6. Lafontan M, Barbe P, Galitzky J, Tavernier G, Langin D *et al.* Adrenergic regulation of adipocyte metabolism. Hum Reprod. 1997;12 Suppl 1:6-20

7. Bui LT, Nguyen DT, Ambrose PJ. Blood pressure and heart rate effects following a single dose of bitter orange. Ann Pharmacother. 2006;40(1):53-7. Epub 2005 Nov 29

8. Hofstetter R, Kreuder J, von Bernuth G. [The effect of oxedrine on the left ventricle and peripheral vascular resistance] [Article in German] Arzneimittelforschung. 1985;35(12):1844-6

9. Greenway F, de Jonge-Levitan L, Martin C, Roberts A, Grundy I, Parker C. Dietary herbal supplements with phenylephrine for weight loss. J Med Food. 2006;9(4):572-8

10. Bent S, Padula A, Neuhaus J. Safety and efficacy of citrus aurantium for weight loss. Am J Cardiol. 2004;94(10):1359-61

11. Haaz S, Fontaine KR, Cutter G, Limdi N, Perumean-Chaney S, Allison DB. Citrus aurantium and synephrine alkaloids in the treatment of overweight and obesity: an update. Obes Rev. 2006;7(1):79-88

12. Preuss HG, DiFerdinando D, Bagchi M, Bagchi D. Citrus aurantium as a thermogenic, weight-reduction replacement for ephedra: an overview. J Med. 2002;33(1-4):247-64

13. Nykamp DL, Fackih MN, Compton AL. Possible association of acute lateral-wall myocardial infarction and bitter orange supplement. Ann Pharmacother. 2004;38(5):812-6. Epub 2004 Mar 16

14. Gange CA, Madias C, Felix-Getzik EM, Weintraub AR, Estes NA 3rd. Variant angina associated with bitter

orange in a dietary supplement. Mayo Clin Proc. 2006;81(4):545-8

15. Nasir JM, Durning SJ, Ferguson M, Barold HS, Haigney MC. Exercise-induced syncope associated with QT prolongation and ephedra-free Xenadrine. Mayo Clin Proc. 2004;79(8):1059-62

16. Firenzuoli F, Gori L, Galapai C. Adverse reaction to an adrenergic herbal extract (Citrus aurantium). Phytomedicine. 2005;12(3):247-8

17. Holmes RO Jr, Tavee J. Vasospasm and stroke attributable to ephedra-free xenadrine: case report. Mil Med. 2008;173(7):708-10

18. Suzuki O, Matsumoto T, Oya M, Katsumata Y. Oxidation of synephrine by type A and type B monoamine oxidase. Experientia. 1979;35(10):1283-4

19. Malhotra S, Bailey DG, Paine MF, Watkins PB. Seville orange juice-felodipine interaction: comparison with dilute grapefruit juice and involvement of furocoumarins. Clin Pharmacol Ther. 2001;69(1):14-23

20. Edwards DJ, Bernier SM. Naringin and naringenin are not the primary CYP3A inhibitors in grapefruit juice. Life Sci. 1996;59(13):1025-30

Tribulus Terrestris

Other names

Caltrop
Cat's head
Devil's horn
Devil's weed
Protodioscin
Protodioscine
Puncturevine
R = glucose : ramnose (2:1) - 26-0-beta-1-glucopiranosil, 22-hydroxifurost-5-en-3-beta, 26-diol, 3-0-beta-diglucoramnoside

Star rating

2

What is it?

A plant of the genus Tribulus and the family Zygophyllaceae which grows throughout Africa, temperate and tropical regions of Asia, Australia, Europe and the United States. In the USA it is classified as a noxious weed in several states (1).

Tribulus has been used in traditional folk medicine as an aphrodisiac.

Claimed benefits

Increases testosterone levels.

Mode of Action

Tribulus is claimed to increase luteinizing hormone (LH)

output from the pituitary gland which in turn stimulates the Leydig cells in the testes to produce more testosterone.

It is believed that steroidal saponins found in Tribulus are responsible for this effect and in particular the furostanol bisglycoside called protodioscin (sometimes spelled protodioscine) which has the structural formula R = glucose : ramnose (2:1)- 26-o-beta-1-glucopiranosil, 22-hydroxifurost-5-en-3-beta, 26-diol, 3-o-beta-diglucoramnoside is held to be the main active component (2) (3).

Effectiveness

Tribulus first came to attention as a supplement to raise testosterone levels following experiments performed in the 1980's by the Bulgarian pharmaceutical company Sopharma. Tribulus had been used as a traditional Bulgarian folk remedy for infertility and Sopharma carried out trials to test it as a treatment for this. Most of the Sopharma research was not published in medical journals, however some details are given on the company's website.

According to Sopharma, a standardized extract of Tribulus (marketed as Tribestan ® by Sopharma) was given to 8 healthy males at a dose of 250 mg, three times daily for 5 days. This produced an average increase in LH levels of 186% and an increase in testosterone levels of 40%. FSH levels were unaffected. In women, FSH and estradiol serum concentrations were elevated by the preparation while testosterone was only mildly raised (4).

Unfortunately although subsequent studies showed a testosterone increasing effect of Tribulus in animals, the human results have never been replicated in independent studies outside Sopharma.

For example in tests on rats and rams oral Tribulus supplementation has been shown to increase testosterone levels (2) (5).

Notwithstanding in humans no effect has been seen. In a Bulgarian study consisting of 21 healthy males (6), an Australian study on 22 elite male rugby players (7) and an American study of 20 males performing resistance training 3 days a week (8) Tribulus supplementation produced no increase in testosterone levels.

The results of tests for improvements in body composition and exercise performance have been equally disappointing. In a study involving 15 males undertaking an 8 week resistance training program and randomized to receive either Tribulus or a placebo, no improvement in body composition or exercise performance was seen in the Tribulus group (9).

Similarly, in the studies mentioned above (6) (7) involving resistance training males and elite rugby players undertaking resistance training, no differences in strength and fat free mass were noted between the Tribulus and placebo groups.

The differences in results between the original Bulgarian research and later studies is disappointing. A possible reason for the difference in results could be differences in the composition of the Tribulus used. Bulgarian Tribulus may contain a different profile of active components to Tribulus grown under different conditions in other geographical locations. Sopharma itself states that Tribestan ® is standardized to contain a minimum of 45% of the active component protodioscin. A review of the labels of the majority of other Tribulus supplements on the market reveals that while many state they contain a standardized amount of saponins, usually 40% or 45%, none specifically state that they are standardized for protodioscin content.

While this may offer a possible explanation, until the benefits of Tribulus supplementation on human testosterone levels have been replicated by researchers outside Sopharma the use of Tribulus to increase testosterone levels cannot be recommended. For those who do wish to use Tribulus it would be sensible to use a formulation standardized specifically for protodioscin content.

Commonly used dosages

Tribulus is sold both in combination with other ingredients, usually in testosterone boosting products, and as a stand alone supplement.

As a stand alone supplement it is sold in capsules from 500mg to 1000mg with a recommended intakes ranging from 1000mg to 2000mg a day.

The recommended dose of Tribestan ® is 1 or 2 tablets of 250 mg 3 times a day with meals (10).

Safety

Tribulus has been reported to increase prostate weight in rats and so has a theoretical potential to aggravate conditions such as benign prostatic hyperplasia (BPH) and prostate cancer (11).

Interactions

Tribulus has been reported to have a blood glucose lowering effect in mice and so may theoretically potentiate the effect of diabetic medications which lower blood sugar levels. This would increase the risk of hypoglycemic episodes. Tribulus should be used with caution by diabetics (12).

References

1. United States Department of Agriculture, Agricultural Research Service, Germplasm Resources Information Network [online] at http://www.ars-grin.gov/cgi-bin/npgs/html/taxon.pl?100965
2. El-Tantawy WH, Temraz A, El-Gindi OD. Free serum testosterone level in male rats treated with Tribulus alatus extracts. Int Braz J Urol. 2007;33(4):554-8; discussion 558-9
3. Bulgarian Pharmaceutical Group Ltd, BiogenicStimulants.com, D.Obreshkova, T.Pangarova, S.Milkov and D.Dinchev. Comparative Analytical Investigation Of Tribulus Terrestris Preparations, Publication in Pharmacia, vol. XLV, bk. 2/1998, 11. Sopharma Ltd. [online] at http://www.tribestan.com/tribulus-comparative-investigations.phtml
4. Bulgarian Pharmaceutical Group Ltd, BiogenicStimulants.com, S. Milanov, A. Maleeva, M. Taskov. Tribestan Effect On The Concentration of Some Hormones In The Serum of Healthy Subjects. RIRR - Radioisotope and Radioimmunological Laboratory, Sofia Chemical Pharmaceutical Research Institute. [online] at http://www.bpg.bg/tribestan/tribulus_424_007.phtml
5. Dimitrov M, Georgiev P, Vitanov S. [Use of tribestan on rams with sexual disorders]. [Article in Bulgarian] Vet Med Nauki. 1987;24(5):102-10
6. Neychev VK, Mitev VI. The aphrodisiac herb Tribulus terrestris does not influence the androgen production in young men. J Ethnopharmacol. 2005;101(1-3):319-23
7. Rogerson S, Riches CJ, Jennings C, Weatherby RP, Meir RA, Marshall-Gradisnik SM. The effect of five weeks of Tribulus terrestris supplementation on muscle strength

and body composition during preseason training in elite rugby league players. J Strength Cond Res. 2007;21(2):348-53

8. Brown GA, Vukovich MD, Reifenrath TA, Uhl NL, Parsons KA *et al.* Effects of anabolic precursors on serum testosterone concentrations and adaptations to resistance training in young men. Int J Sport Nutr Exerc Metab. 2000;10(3):340-59

9. Antonio J, Uelmen J, Rodriguez R, Earnest C. The effects of Tribulus terrestris on body composition and exercise performance in resistance-trained males. Int J Sport Nutr Exerc Metab. 2000;10(2):208-15

10. Bulgarian Pharmaceutical Group Ltd, BiogenicStimulants.com, Tribestan, Documentation for Registration. [online] at http://www.bpg.bg/tribestan/tribulus_424_012.phtml

11. Gauthaman K, Adaikan PG, Prasad RN. Aphrodisiac properties of Tribulus Terrestris extract (Protodioscin) in normal and castrated rats. Life Sci. 2002;71(12):1385-96

12. Li M, Qu W, Wang Y, Wan H, Tian C. [Hypoglycemic effect of saponin from Tribulus terrestris]. [Article in Chinese] Zhong Yao Cai. 2002;25(6):420-2

Uva ursi

Other names

Arbutin
Arctostaphylos uva ursi
Bear's grape
Bearberry
Common bearberry

Star rating

2

What is it?

A herb in the genus Arctostaphylos used in traditional medicine as a remedy for urinary tract infections. It produces red berries and grows in alpine forests of various regions, including North America, Europe, Siberia and the Himalayas (1).

Claimed benefits

Diuretic.

Mode of Action

The active principle in Uva ursi responsible for the diuretic effect is the phenol glycoside arbutin (2). Exactly how arbutin functions as a diuretic is unknown.

Effectiveness

The ability of Uva ursi to act as a diuretic only appears to have been confirmed in a single study on rats (3).

Commonly used dosages

Uva ursi is included in sport supplements in a wide range of amounts from 200mg up to 1500mg. Sometimes labels state that the extract is standardized for arbutin content, usually 20 – 30%.

The lack of human studies makes it difficult to comment on the effectiveness of these doses.

For urinary tract infections the recommended dose is 2 - 4 g per day, standardized for 400 - 800 mg of arbutin (1).

Safety

Uva ursi is approved by the German Commission E for the treatment of urinary tract infections for periods up to 2 weeks. Its use longer than 2 weeks is not recommended. This is because Uva ursi is hydrolyzed in the gut to hydroquinone and there is concern that long term exposure to hydroquinone may cause cancer (4).

Hydroquinone can also inhibit melanin production. Melanin is the pigment which gives the skin and eyes their color. There is a report of a woman suffering eye damage (Bull's eye maculopathy) due to reduced retinal melanin production after taking Uva ursi for 3 years (5).

Interactions

None known.

References

1. University of Maryland Medical Center, Uva ursi, [online] at http://www.umm.edu/altmed/articles/uva-ursi-000278.htm
2. Kar A. Pharmacognosy and Pharmacobiotechnology. New Delhi; New Age International (P) Limited: 2003
3. Beaux D, Fleurentin J, Mortier F. Effect of extracts of Orthosiphon stamineus Benth, Hieracium pilosella L., Sambucus nigra L. and Arctostaphylos uva-ursi (L.) Spreng. in rats. Phytother Res. 1999;13(3):222-5
4. Yarnell E. Botanical medicines for the urinary tract. World J Urol. 2002;20(5):285-93. Epub 2002 Oct 17
5. Wang L, Del Priore LV. Bull's-eye maculopathy secondary to herbal toxicity from uva ursi. Am J Ophthalmol. 2004;137(6):1135-7

Whey protein

Other names

Milk soluble proteins

Star rating

5

What is it?

A protein derived from milk.

Milk contains 3.3% protein containing all 8 essential amino acids. This protein is actually composed of two kinds of protein 82% casein and 18% whey. Both of these in turn are made up of various components. Whey is composed of about 50% ß-lactoglobulin, 20% α-lactalbumin and the balance made up of blood serum albumin, lactoferrin, transferrin, various immunoglobulins and other minor proteins. Casein is composed of 4 different caseins which all have their own amino acid structure; α-s1, α-s2 , ß, and kappa-casein (1).

After the fat is removed from milk to leave skimmed milk, this can be subjected to various further processes to extract its casein and whey protein content.

Ultrafiltration removes the lactose (milk carbohydrate content) from the milk leaving behind a milk protein concentrate (MPC) which contains the same proportions of micellar casein and whey as natural milk, i.e. 82% casein and 18% whey.

Microfiltration is then used to separate the casein and whey constituents to produce either pure micellar casein or whey. Casein and whey protein have a greatly differing amino acid composition. Whey contains higher concentrations of the sulphur containing amino acids methionine and cysteine, lysine, threonine, and tryptophan.

Commercially sold whey supplements are usually either whey protein concentrate, whey isolate or whey hydrolysate or combinations of the three. Whey concentrate usually contains around 80% protein with the other 20% made up of lactose and fat from milk. Whey isolate has been further filtered to increase its purity and contains at least 90% protein. Whey hydrolysate is whey which has been partially broken down into smaller amino acids by enzymes. This allows the body to absorb it even faster, however the process leaves it with an unpleasant bitter taste so when hydrolysate is used in supplements it is usually mixed with other forms of whey.

Claimed benefits

Anabolic effect via increased protein synthesis, particularly when taken post workout.

Mode of Action

Whey protein exerts its anabolic effect both through its composition and its speed of absorption.

Whey protein and particularly the β-lactoglobulin fraction is a rich source of branched chain amino acids (BCAA). β-lactoglobulin is composed of 14.5% of the BCAA leucine which acts as a signalling molecule to increase protein synthesis and skeletal muscle size by triggering a cell signalling pathway called mTORC1.

Furthermore there is some evidence that peptide bound BCAA derived from whey protein elicit a greater increase in muscle protein synthesis than free form BCAA supplements.

The speed of absorption of whey protein is a further important factor. Whey protein remains soluble in the stomach and exits quickly undigested in liquid form. It then undergoes digestion by pancreatic enzymes and is absorbed in the lower part of the small intestine. Whey therefore delivers amino acids at a fast rate and high concentration which causes a greater muscle protein synthesis response than other slower digested forms of protein (2) (3) (4).

Effectiveness

There is overwhelming evidence that protein both stimulates muscle protein synthesis under resting conditions and enhances muscle adaptation to the effect of physical exercise and resistance training. Protein supplementation in combination with resistance training increases muscle fibre thickness and lean body mass when compared to fasting or carbohydrate supplements (2).

The beneficial effect of protein is greatest when it is consumed immediately before or immediately following exercise since there appears to be a "window of opportunity" following exercise during which uptake of amino acids and glucose into muscles is enhanced (2) (5).

In addition whey protein added to carbohydrate improves post exercise muscle glycogen replenishment (6) (7) which may be due to the fact that whey increases the insulin response to carbohydrate (2).

The superiority of whey protein over other protein sources for increasing the rate of muscle protein synthesis has been seen in various studies. For example in one recent study whey was shown to increase protein synthesis 93% and 18% more than casein and soy at rest, and 122% and 31% more than casein and soy following exercise (8).

Another study found that whey protein increased net protein synthesis by 68% while casein increased it by 31% (9).

However the increased protein synthesis induced by whey has a short duration of approximately 3 to 4 hours so it must be taken frequently to maintain its effect (9) (10).

Over the long term, in a study involving 13 recreational bodybuilders undertaking a 10 week resistance training program and supplementing their diet with either casein or whey protein (at 1.5g/kg of bodyweight per day) the group supplementing with whey protein gained five times more lean mass than the casein group and significantly greater strength gains (11).

Commonly used dosages

Commercial whey protein supplements typically recommend an intake of 25g two or three times a day.

This seems to be supported by the available evidence which suggests that although as little as 10g of whey can stimulate muscle protein synthesis, amounts higher than approximately 30g do not seem to have any greater effect. In other words there is a plateau effect beyond which consuming more than 30g of whey does not provide any additional benefit (2).

For endurance sports consuming carbohydrate and protein at a ratio of 4:1 increases endurance performance during both acute exercise and subsequent bouts of endurance exercise (12).

Safety

No known safety issues.

Interactions

None known.

References

1. Cornell University, Milk Protein [online] at http://www.milkfacts.info/Milk%20Composition/protein.htm
2. Hulmi JJ, Lockwood CM, Stout JR. Effect of protein/essential amino acids and resistance training on skeletal muscle hypertrophy: A case for whey protein. Nutr Metab (Lond). 2010;17;7:51

3. Laplante M, Sabatini DM. mTOR signaling at a glance. J Cell Sci. 2009 Oct;122(Pt 20):3589-94
4. Mahé S, Roos N, Benamouzig R, Davin L, Luengo C *et al.* Gastrojejunal kinetics and the digestion of [15N]beta-lactoglobulin and casein in humans: the influence of the nature and quantity of the protein. Am J Clin Nutr. 1996;63(4):546-52
5. Esmarck B, Andersen JL, Olsen S, Richter EA, Mizuno M, Kjaer M. Timing of postexercise protein intake is important for muscle hypertrophy with resistance training in elderly humans. J Physiol. 2001;535(Pt 1):301-11
6. Jentjens R, Jeukendrup A. Determinants of post-exercise glycogen synthesis during short-term recovery. Sports Med. 2003;33(2):117-44
7. van Loon LJ, Saris WH, Kruijshoop M, Wagenmakers AJ. Maximizing postexercise muscle glycogen synthesis: carbohydrate supplementation and the application of amino acid or protein hydrolysate mixtures. Am J Clin Nutr. 2000;72(1):106-11
8. Tang JE, Moore DR, Kujbida GW, Tarnopolsky MA, Phillips SM. Ingestion of whey hydrolysate, casein, or soy protein isolate: effects on mixed muscle protein synthesis at rest and following resistance exercise in young men. J Appl Physiol. 2009;107(3):987-92. Epub 2009 Jul 9
9. Boirie Y, Dangin M, Gachon P, Vasson MP, Maubois JL, Beaufrère B. Slow and fast dietary proteins differently modulate postprandial protein accretion. Proc Natl Acad Sci U S A. 1997;94(26):14930-5
10. Lacroix M, Bos C, Léonil J, Airinei G, Luengo C *et al.* Compared with casein or total milk protein, digestion of milk soluble proteins is too rapid to sustain the anabolic postprandial amino acid requirement. Am J Clin Nutr. 2006;84(5):1070-9
11. Cribb PJ, Williams AD, Carey MF, Hayes A. The effect of whey isolate and resistance training on strength, body

composition, and plasma glutamine. Int J Sport Nutr Exerc Metab. 2006;16(5):494-509
12. Kerksick C, Harvey T, Stout J, Campbell B, Wilborn C *et al*. International Society of Sports Nutrition position stand: nutrient timing. J Int Soc Sports Nutr. 2008;5:17

Yohimbe / Yohimbine

Other names

(16α,17α)-17-Hydroxyyohimban-16-carboxylic acid methyl ester
Antagonil
Aphrodine
Corynine
Johimbi
Pausinystalia yohimbe
Quebrachine
Rauwolfia
Yohimbine hydrochloride

Star rating

3

What is it?

Yohimbe (Corynanthe johimbe) is an African evergreen tree the bark of which contains less than 10% of the indole alkaloid yohimbine which is an α2 receptor antagonist. Yohimbine is also found in Rubiaceae and Rauwolfia serpentina (1) (2).

Supplements may contain either the whole bark or the

isolated yohimbine component. Yohimbine is also available in some countries as a prescription medication for erectile dysfunction.

Claimed benefits

Fat loss.

Yohimbe is claimed to be especially effective at aiding loss of fat from the hips and thighs in women and the stomach in men.

Mode of Action

Lipolysis (burning of body fat for energy) is regulated by the presence of receptors on fat cells which react to the presence of the fat burning hormones epinephrine (adrenaline) and norepinephrine (noradrenaline).

At low concentrations of epinephrine and norepinephrine (such as at rest) the α2 receptors are preferentially activated and these receptors inhibit lipolysis. However at higher concentrations (such as during exercise) the β1 and β2 receptors become activated and these activate lipolysis. So it can be seen that anything which either blocks the action of α2 receptors or increases the action of β1 and β2 receptors will promote fat loss (3).

It is also of interest that the way these receptors control the rate of lipolysis can vary by location on the body and between the sexes, probably due to the proportion of α2 receptors and β1 and β2 receptors present. During exercise lipolysis is greater in abdominal fat than in thigh and gluteal fat and this difference is greater in women. This may explain why women tend to accumulate more fat on the thighs and buttocks than men, but less fat on the abdomen (4) (5).

Yohimbine acts as an α2 receptor antagonist which means it blocks the action of this receptor. This causes two effects, firstly it reduces the inhibitory action of fat cell α2 receptors and increases the amount of fat burned at rest.

Secondly, blocking α2 receptors in the sympathetic nervous system causes an increase in the amount of norepinephrine released which then causes an increase in lipolysis via activation of β1 and β2 receptors (6) (7).

Of the two mechanisms it seems that the increase in norepinephrine is the most important action of yohimbine accounting for at least 70% of its lipolytic effect (6) (8).

Effectiveness

In studies, healthy non obese men and women who were given 0.2mg/kg had an average increase in norepinephrine levels of 100% for the women and 50% for the men after oral yohimbine administration, and induced lipolysis for a minimum of 240 minutes (as long as was measured in the study). There was no significant effect on plasma glucose, insulin levels, heart rate or blood pressure (6) (7).

However studies measuring actual fat loss have had mixed results. In one study of 20 obese women given either 20mg of yohimbine/day or a placebo for 3 weeks the yohimbine group had an average weight loss of 3.55kg compared to only 2.21kg for the placebo group (9).

In another study involving 20 professional soccer players taking 20mg/day for 21 days, fat mass was approximately 2% lower in the yohimbine group compared to placebo (10)

Nevertheless, in another study of 19 obese volunteers given 18mg yohimbine/day for 8 weeks there was no difference in weight loss compared to placebo (11).

Similarly in a study of 47 men given 43mg yohimbine/day for 6 months there was no difference in body weight or fat distribution as measured both by waist-to-hip ratio and by CT scan compared to the placebo group (12).

Commonly used dosages

Yohimbine is usually included as part of a proprietary formulation in commercial sport supplement preparations with the exact quantity of the substance not listed in the ingredients.

It can also be bought as a stand alone supplement both as yohimbine and yohimbe bark.

Amounts of around 20mg/day have been used in most of the studies mentioned above.

Yohimbine should not be taken with food since $\alpha 2$ antagonism in the presence of food augments pancreatic insulin secretion which counteracts any lipolytic effects. However this effect does not occur if yohimbine is taken without food (8).

Safety

Records from the California Poison Control System show that between 2000 and 2006 238 adverse events associated with yohimbine use were reported. Many of these were associated with severe outcomes likely to require management in a health facility. The most common adverse events were gastrointestinal distress, tachycardia, anxiety, and high blood pressure (13).

Interactions

Yohimbine has a major interaction with a class of antidepressants called monoamine oxidase inhibitors (MAOI's) and can increase the effects and side effects of these medicines.

It also interacts with tricyclic antidepressants and may cause heart problems if taken together. You should consult your doctor if you are on any kind of antidepressants before taking yohimbine to check it is safe.

Because yohimbine may increase your blood pressure it can interfere with any blood pressure medication you may be taking such as captopril, losartan, diuretics etc.

The medications naloxone and phenothiazines and stimulant drugs such as pseudoephedrine (Sudafed) may increase the undesirable side effects of yohimbine such as anxiety, tremor, high blood pressure etc.

If you are taking any of these kinds of medicines you should avoid yohimbine (14).

References

1. Medline Plus, Yohimbe [online] at http://www.nlm.nih.gov/medlineplus/druginfo/natural/759.html
2. The Merck Index 14th Ed. New Jersey, Merck & Co. Inc. 2006.
3. Lafontan M, Barbe P, Galitzky J, Tavernier G, Langin D *et al.* Adrenergic regulation of adipocyte metabolism. Hum Reprod. 1997;12 Suppl 1:6-20

4. Arner P, Kriegholm E, Engfeldt P, Bolinder J. Adrenergic regulation of lipolysis in situ at rest and during exercise. J Clin Invest. 1990;85(3):893-8

5. Mauriege P, Galitzky J, Berlan M, Lafontan M. Heterogeneous distribution of beta and alpha-2 adrenoceptor binding sites in human fat cells from various fat deposits: functional consequences. Eur J Clin Invest. 1987;17(2):156-65

6. Berlan M, Galitzky J, Riviere D, Foureau M, Tran MA *et al.* Plasma catecholamine levels and lipid mobilization induced by yohimbine in obese and non-obese women. Int J Obes. 1991;15(5):305-15

7. Galitzky J, Taouis M, Berlan M, Rivière D, Garrigues M, Lafontan M. Alpha 2-antagonist compounds and lipid mobilization: evidence for a lipid mobilizing effect of oral yohimbine in healthy male volunteers. Eur J Clin Invest. 1988;18(6):587-94

8. Lafontan M, Berlan M, Galitzky J, Montastruc JL. Alpha-2 adrenoceptors in lipolysis: alpha 2 antagonists and lipid-mobilizing strategies. Am J Clin Nutr. 1992;55(1 Suppl):219S-227S

9. Kucio C, Jonderko K, Piskorska D. Does yohimbine act as a slimming drug? Isr J Med Sci. 1991;27(10):550-6

10. Ostojic SM. Yohimbine: the effects on body composition and exercise performance in soccer players. Res Sports Med. 2006;14(4):289-99

11. Berlin I, Stalla-Bourdillon A, Thuillier Y, Turpin G, Puech AJ. [Lack of efficacy of yohimbine in the treatment of obesity]. [Article in French] J Pharmacol. 1986;17(3):343-7

12. Sax L. Yohimbine does not affect fat distribution in men. Int J Obes. 1991;15(9):561-5

13. Kearney T, Tu N, Haller C. Adverse drug events associated with yohimbine-containing products: a retrospective review of the California Poison Control

System reported cases. Ann Pharmacother. 2010;44(6):1022-9. Epub 2010 May 4

14. Medline Plus, Yohimbe, Are there interactions with medications? [online] at http://www.nlm.nih.gov/medlineplus/druginfo/natural/759.html#DrugInteractions

ZMA

Other names

None

Star rating

3

What is it?

A patented combination of 30 mg zinc monomethionine aspartate, 450 mg magnesium aspartate, and 10.5 mg of vitamin B-6.

The patent holder is a company called SNAC System Inc.

Claimed benefits

Increases strength, testosterone levels and Insulin-like Growth Factor-I (IGF-I) levels.

Mode of Action

Several studies have shown that high level athletes

frequently become deficient in levels of magnesium and zinc (1) (2) (3).

Magnesium is necessary for various muscle processes such as energy production, oxygen uptake and electrolyte balance. It may also help reduce cortisol levels which can have adverse effects on muscle mass (4) (5).

Likewise zinc is necessary for the activity of several enzymes in energy metabolism and low muscle zinc levels result in reduced muscle endurance capacity (2) (6).

Low zinc levels are also associated with lower testosterone levels (7).

ZMA aims to prevent any of these deficiencies occurring by providing supplemental magnesium and zinc. The vitamin B-6 component is included because it increases the absorption of magnesium and zinc (8) (9).

Effectiveness

Before looking at ZMA itself we will examine prior studies on either magnesium or zinc supplementation alone.

Magnesium supplementation has been shown to have beneficial effects on exercise performance in magnesium-deficient individuals but not in individuals with adequate magnesium status (10).

Likewise, in zinc deficient individuals, zinc supplementation has been shown to improve muscle strength and increase testosterone levels (6) (7) (11).

The patent holders of ZMA conducted a study in which they claimed that when 57 university football players took either

ZMA or a placebo for 7 weeks during the spring practice season, the ZMA group had greater strength gains than the placebo group and had an increase in testosterone levels of 32% and an increase in IGF-1 levels of 3.6% compared to a drop in testosterone of 10% in the placebo group and a drop in IGF-1 of 21.5%.

However the full study has never been published in a scientific journal and when a short abstract (summary) was published in the journal Medicine & Science in Sports & Exercise the claims relating to increases in testosterone and IGF-1 were not included (12).

Studies performed by independent researchers not connected to the patent holder have shown less impressive results.

In one study of 42 men undertaking resistance training 4 days a week and taking either ZMA or a placebo for 8 weeks no differences were found in strength or body composition and ZMA did not increase testosterone levels compared to placebo (13).

In a different study 14 regularly exercising men given ZMA also showed no increase in testosterone levels (14).

Could there be any explanation for the differences in findings? One reason could be differences in the type of sports or exercises undertaken in the studies. Evidence of magnesium and zinc deficiencies has only been observed in professional athletes, those undertaking a high level of constant exercise or sports people who have to make weight categories such as wrestlers and gymnasts. The benefits of zinc and magnesium supplements in all the studies looked at above were only apparent in individuals in these categories or those suffering from dietary deficiencies.

In the patent holders study on ZMA the participants were university level football players undertaking an intensive 8 week training season and there was a significant difference in zinc and magnesium levels between the ZMA and placebo groups.

By contrast in the independent study which found no effect there was no significant difference between zinc and magnesium levels between the two groups.

In conclusion, the benefit from zinc and magnesium supplementation is seen in people with deficiency caused by undertaking intense levels of sporting activity or from dietary deficiency. Individuals with good nutrition and undertaking intermittent exercise such as a 4 day a week weight training program as in the independent study are unlikely to have zinc or magnesium deficiencies and are unlikely to get any benefit from supplementation.

Commonly used dosages

The recommended serving of ZMA contains 30mg of zinc, 450mg of magnesium and 10.5mg of vitamin B6.

In the US the Reference Daily Intake amounts set by the FDA are 15mg for zinc, 400mg for magnesium and 2mg for vitamin B6.

In the EU the Recommended Daily Allowances are 15mg for zinc, 300mg for magnesium and 2mg for vitamin B6.

Safety

No known safety issues at the recommended doses although zinc, magnesium and vitamin B6 can pose health risks if taken in excess. Do not exceed the recommended doses and exercise care if combining with other vitamin or mineral supplements.

The US daily upper safe levels for supplements of these nutrients are zinc 40mg, magnesium 350mg and vitamin B6 100mg (15).

The EU daily upper intake levels are 25mg zinc, magnesium 250mg and vitamin B6 25mg (16).

Note: The US upper limits are for supplements only. The EU upper limits are for combined intake from food and supplements. Bizarrely the EU upper limit for magnesium of 250mg is *below* the EU RDA of 300mg. The EU upper limits have been widely criticized.

Interactions

Both magnesium and zinc can inhibit absorption of quinolone antibiotics such as ciprofloxacin and tetracycline antibiotics, you should separate taking zinc or magnesium and antibiotics by at least 3 hours (17) (18) (19).

Zinc can also interfere with the absorption of the medicine penicillamine, take them separated by at least 3 hours (20).

Magnesium supplements should be avoided by anyone taking a potassium sparing diuretic such as spironolactone (aldactone) as this could lead to dangerously high magnesium levels.

References

1.   Haralambie G. Serum zinc in athletes in training. Int J Sports Med. 1981;2(3):135-8

2. Cordova A, Alvarez-Mon M. Behaviour of zinc in physical exercise: a special reference to immunity and fatigue. Neurosci Biobehav Rev. 1995;19(3):439-45

3. Singh A, Day BA, DeBolt JE, Trostmann UH, Bernier LL, Deuster PA. Magnesium, zinc, and copper status of US Navy SEAL trainees. Am J Clin Nutr. 1989;49(4):695-700

4. Nielsen FH, Lukaski HC. Update on the relationship between magnesium and exercise. Magnes Res. 2006;19(3):180-9

5. Wilborn CD, Kerksick CM, Campbell BI, Taylor LW, Marcello BM *et al*. Effects of Zinc Magnesium Aspartate (ZMA) Supplementation on Training Adaptations and Markers of Anabolism and Catabolism. J Int Soc Sports Nutr. 2004;1(2):12-20

6. Van Loan MD, Sutherland B, Lowe NM, Turnlund JR, King JC. The effects of zinc depletion on peak force and total work of knee and shoulder extensor and flexor muscles. Int J Sport Nutr. 1999;9(2):125-35

7. Prasad AS, Mantzoros CS, Beck FW, Hess JW, Brewer GJ. Zinc status and serum testosterone levels of healthy adults. Nutrition. 1996;12(5):344-8

8. Wischnik A, Schroll A, Kollmer WE, Berg D, Wischnik B *et al*. [Magnesium aspartate as a cardioprotective agent and adjuvant in tocolysis with betamimetics. Animal experiments on the kinetics and calcium antagonist action of orally administered magnesium aspartate with special reference to simultaneous vitamin B administration]. [Article in German] Z Geburtshilfe Perinatol. 1982;186(6):326-34

9. Evans GW, Johnson EC. Effect of iron, vitamin B-6 and picolinic acid on zinc absorption in the rat. J Nutr. 1981;111(1):68-75

10. Nielsen FH, Lukaski HC. Update on the relationship between magnesium and exercise. Magnes Res. 2006;19(3):180-9

11. Kilic M, Baltaci AK, Gunay M, Gökbel H, Okudan N, Cicioglu I. The effect of exhaustion exercise on thyroid hormones and testosterone levels of elite athletes receiving oral zinc. Neuro Endocrinol Lett. 2006;27(1-2):247-52

12. Brilla LR, Conte V. Effects of Zinc-Magnesium (Zma) Supplementation on Muscle Attributes of Football Players. Medicine & Science in Sports & Exercise 1999;35(5):S123

13. Wilborn CD, Kerksick CM, Campbell BI, Taylor LW, Marcello BM et al. Effects of Zinc Magnesium Aspartate (ZMA) Supplementation on Training Adaptations and Markers of Anabolism and Catabolism. J Int Soc Sports Nutr. 2004;1(2):12-20

14. Koehler K, Parr MK, Geyer H, Mester J, Schänzer W. Serum testosterone and urinary excretion of steroid hormone metabolites after administration of a high-dose zinc supplement. Eur J Clin Nutr. 2009;63(1):65-70. Epub 2007 Sep 19

15. Office of Dietary Supplements. National Institutes of Health. Vitamin and Mineral Supplements Fact Sheets. [online] at http://ods.od.nih.gov/factsheets/list-VitaminsMinerals/

16. European Food Safety Authority. Tolerable Upper Intake Levels for Vitamins and Minerals by the Scientific Panel on Dietetic products, nutrition and allergies (NDA) and Scientific Committee on Food (SCF). [online] at http://www.efsa.europa.eu/en/home/oldsc/ndaintakevitaminsminerals.htm

17. Lomaestro BM, Bailie GR. Absorption interactions with fluoroquinolones. 1995 update. Drug Saf. 1995;12(5):314-33

18. Andersson KE, Bratt L, Dencker H, Kamme C, Lanner E. Inhibition of tetracycline absorption by zinc. Eur J Clin Pharmacol. 1976;10:59-62

19. Sompolinsky D, Samra Z. Influence of magnesium and manganese on some biological and physical properties of tetracycline. J Bacteriol. 1972;110(2):468-76
20. Mery C, Delrieu F, Ghozlan R, Saporta L, Simon F *et al.* Controlled trial of D-penicillamine in rheumatoid arthritis. Dose effect and the role of zinc. Scand J Rheumatol. 1976;5(4):241-7

Glossary of terms

Adipocytes – fat cells

Adipose – fat tissue

Aerobic exercise – low or moderate intensity exercise such as running, cycling etc performed at a rate where the body is capable of supplying sufficient oxygen to the muscles

Agonist – a substance which can be naturally produced in the body such as a hormone or supplied from outside such as drug which acts on a cellular receptor to produce a certain effect or response.

Anabolic – a metabolic process producing growth or synthesis of tissue, usually refers to muscle growth.

Anaerobic exercise – high intensity exercise such as weight lifting and sprinting etc where oxygen is used faster then the body is able to replace it.

Anatagonist - a substance which can be naturally produced in the body such as a hormone or supplied from outside such as drug which acts on a cellular receptor to block its effect or response.

Arrhythmia – an abnormal heart rhythm.

Catabolic – a metabolic process producing breakdown of tissue or muscle.

Cognition – mental processes such as thinking, reasoning, remembering etc

Cortisol – a hormone produced in the body and increased by stress, injury etc. It plays an important role in reducing inflammation but also has catabolic effects on muscle and can promote fat deposition.

Diuretic – a substance or process which increases loss of water from the body by increasing the amount of urine produced.

Endogenous – refers to anything produced naturally within the body.

Enzyme – a substance which initiates or speeds up a chemical reaction

Exogenous – refers to anything which is supplied to the body artificially e.g anabolic steroids are exogenous hormones.

Follicle stimulating hormone – a hormone produced in the pituitary gland which in women stimulates the growth of follicles in the ovaries and in men stimulates the testicles to produce sperm.

HDL – high density lipoprotein, the "good" type of cholesterol.

Hepatic – refers to any process involving the liver.

Hepatotoxin - a substance which is poisonous to liver cells.

Hyperglycemia – a state in which levels of sugar in the blood are abnormally high.

Hyperlipidemia – the condition of having abnormally high cholesterol.

Hypoglycemia - a state in which levels of sugar in the blood are abnormally low.

Hypothalamus – a part of the brain involved in the control of metabolism and which controls the pituitary gland.

In vitro – a test or experiment using cells or tissue.

In vivo – a test or experiment using live animals or human beings.

Isomers – substances composed of the same elements but whose atoms have different arrangement which alters their properties.

LDL – low density lipoprotein, the "bad" type of cholesterol.

Lipogenesis – the formation and accumulation of fat.

Lipolysis – the metabolic process of burning fat for energy.

Luteinizing hormone - a hormone produced in the pituitary gland which in women stimulates ovulation and in men stimulates the testicles to produce testosterone.

Phytoestrogen - a group of substances which occur naturally in plants which have a structural similarity to the hormone estrogen and so can have estrogen like effects in humans.

Pituitary gland – a small gland in the brain just below the hypothalamus which produces the hormones luteinizing hormone and follicle stimulating hormone among others.

Placebo – a substance which has no physiological or pharmacological effect in the body used as a control when testing other compounds.

Proprietary formulation – a unique mixture of substances developed by a particular company for its supposed effect or benefit. The exact quantities of individual substances in proprietary formulations are usually kept secret.

Randomised double blind trial – An experiment where the subjects are assigned to receive either a real treatment or a placebo at random and neither the subjects themselves nor the experimenters know who has received the real treatment or the placebo until the end of the trial.

Receptor – a molecular receptor located on a cell to which a signalling molecule such as a hormone or drug may attach producing a specific effect or response in the cell.

Systematic review – a review and analysis of all the research which has been carried out on a particular topic to try and reach a conclusion on it.

Testes – the testicles.

Thermogenesis – the process of heat production in organisms.

Vasoconstriction – the narrowing of blood vessels caused by constriction of their muscular lining.

Expanded Contents

β-Guanidinopropionic acid – see guanidinoproprionic acid

β-Hydroxy β-Methylbutyrate Monohydrate – see HMB

β-Hydroxy-β-Methylbutyric Acid – see HMB

(β-hydroxyethyl)trimethylammonium – see choline

[(3R,4aR,5S,6S,6aS,10S,10aR,10bS)-3-ethenyl-6,10,10b-trihydroxy-3,4a,7, 7,10a-pentamethyl-1-oxo-5,6,6a,8,9,10-hexahydro-2H-benzo[f]chromen-5-yl] acetate – see forskolin

1-(4-hydroxyphenyl)-2-methylaminoethanol – see synephrine

1-(p-hydroxyphenyl)-2-aminoethanol – see octopamine

1,3,7-trimethyl-2,6-dioxopurine – see caffeine

1,3,7-trimethylpurine-2,6-dione – see caffeine

1,3,7-Trimethylxanthine – see caffeine

1,3-Dimethylamylamine – see geranamine

1,3-Dimethylamylamine HCL – see geranamine

1,3-Dimethylpentylamine – see geranamine

10-hydroxy-2,4a,6a,6b,9,9,12a-heptamethyl-13-oxo-3,4,5,6,6a,7,8,8a,10, 11,12,14b-dodecahydro-1H-picene-2-carboxylic acid – see glycyrrhetinic acid

11,20-dihydroxyecdysone – see ecdysteroids

15,16-dodecahydrocyclopenta[a]phenanthren-17-one – see DHEA

17beta-acetoxy-8,13-epoxy-1alpha,6beta,9alpha-trihydroxylabd-14-en-11-one – see forskolin

1-Amino-4-guanidobutane – see agmatine

1-Carboxy-N,N,N-trimethylmethanaminium inner salt – see betaine

2-(10-hydroxydecyl)-5,6-dimethoxy-3-methylcyclohexa-2,5-diene-1,4-dione – see idebenone

2-(3,4-Dihydroxyphenyl)ethyl (2S-(2alpha,3E,4beta))-3-ethylidene-2-(beta-D-glucopyranosyloxy)-3,4-dihydro-5-(methoxycarbonyl)-2H-pyran-4-acetate – see oleuropein

2-(4-aminobutyl)guanidine – see agmatine

2,3-dimethoxy-5-methyl-6-(10-hydroxydecyl)-1,4-benzoquinone – see idebenone

2-[carbamimidoyl(methyl)amino]acetic acid – see creatine monohydrate

20 Beta-Hydroxyecdysterone – see ecdysteroids

20E – see ecdysteroids

20-hydroxyecdysone – see ecdysteroids

22:23-dihydrostigmasterol – see beta sitosterol

24β-ethyl-Δ5-cholesten-3β-ol – see beta sitosterol

2-Amino-4-methylhexane – see geranamine

2-Aminopentanoic acid – see norvaline

2-Aminovaleric acid – see norvaline

2-Carboxyethylamine – see beta alanine

2-hexanamine, 4-methyl- – see geranamine

2-Hexanamine, 4-methyl- (9CI) – see geranamine

2-hydroxyethyl(trimethyl)azanium – see choline

2-Hydroxy-N,N,N-trimethylethanaminium – see choline

2-ketoglutarate – see alpha-ketoglutarate

2-ketoglutaric acid – see alpha-ketoglutarate

2-Oxoglutamate – see alpha-ketoglutarate

2-oxoglutarate – see alpha-ketoglutarate

2-oxoglutarate(2-) – see alpha-ketoglutarate

2-oxoglutaric acid – see alpha-ketoglutarate

2-oxopentanedioate – see alpha-ketoglutarate

3 beta-acetoxy-androst-5-ene-7,17-dione – see 7-keto-DHEA

3-(*1H*-Indol-3-ylmethyl)-*1H*-indole – see DIM

3-(diaminomethylideneamino)propanoic acid – see guanidinoproprionic acid

3,3'-Diindolylmethane – see DIM

3,3'-Methylenebis-*1H*-indole – see DIM

3,4',5-stilbenetriol – see resveratrol

3,4,8,10-tetrahydroxy-2-(hydroxymethyl)-9-methoxy-3,4,4a,10b-tetrahydropyrano[3,2-c]isochromen-6(2H)-one – see bergenin

3,5,4'-trihydroxystilbene – see resveratrol

3,7-Dihydro-1,3,7-trimethyl-1H-purine-2,6-dione – see caffeine

3-acetyl-7-oxo-dehydroepiandrosterone – see 7-keto-DHEA

3-Aminopropanoate – see beta alanine
3-Aminopropanoic acid – see beta alanine
3-Aminopropionic acid – see beta alanine
3-Aminopropionsaeure – see beta alanine
3-carbamimidamidopropanoic acid – see guanidinoproprionic acid
3-Glycyrrhetinic acid – see glycyrrhetinic acid
3-Guanidinopropanoate – see guanidinoproprionic acid
3-Guanidinopropionic acid – see guanidinoproprionic acid
3-Guanidino-propionic acid – see guanidinoproprionic acid
4-(4-hydroxyphenyl) butan-2-one – see raspberry ketones
4',5,7-trihydroxyflavanone 7-rhamnoglucoside – see naringin
4-[2-(Dimethylamino)ethyl]phenol – see hordenine
4'5-diOH-Flavone-7-rhgluc – see naringin
4-amino-3-phenylbutyric acid – see phenibut
4-Hydroxy-α-[(methylamino)methyl]benzenemethanol – see synephrine
4-Methyl-2-hexanamine – see geranamine
4-Methylhexan-2-amine – see geranamine
5,6-Dihydro-9,10-dimethoxybenzo[g]-1,3-benzodioxolo[5,6-a]quinolizinium – see berberine
5,8,11,14-Eicosatetraenoic acid – see arachidonic acid
5-[(1E)-2-(4-hydroxyphenyl)ethenyl]-1,3-benzenediol – see resveratrol
5-Methyl-7-Methoxy-Isoflavone – see methoxyisoflavone
7 methoxy – see methoxyisoflavone
7,8,13,13a-tetradehydro-9,10-dimethoxy-2,3-(methylenedioxy)berbinium – see berberine
7-[[2-O-(6-Deoxy-α-L-mannopyranosyl)-β-D-glucopyranosyl]oxy]-2,3-dihydro-5-hydroxy-2-(4-hydroxyphenyl)-4H-1-benzopyran-4-one – see naringin
7-keto Dehydroepiandrosterone – see 7-keto-DHEA
7-methoxy-3-phenyl-4H-chromen-4-one – see methoxyisoflavone
7-methoxyisoflavone – see methoxyisoflavone

7-oxo Dehydroepiandrosterone – see 7-keto-DHEA
7-oxo-dehydroepiandrosterone-3-acetate – see 7-keto-DHEA
7-oxo-DHEA – see 7-keto-DHEA
8,13,13b,14-Tetrahydro-14-
methylindolo[2',3':3,4]pyrido[2,1-b]quinazolin-5(7H)-one –
see evodiamine
9,10-Dimethoxy-2,3-(methylenedioxy)-7,8,13,13a-
tetrahydroberbinium – see berberine

α-(Aminomethyl)-4-hydroxybenzenemethanol – see
octopamine
α-(aminomethyl)-p-hydroxybenzyl alcohol – see octopamine
α-dihydrofucosterol – see beta sitosterol
α-phytosterol – see beta sitosterol
β-methylamino-α-(4-hydroxyphenyl)ethyl alcohol – see
synephrine
Δ5-androsten-3β-ol-17-one – see DHEA
Δ5-stigmasten-3β-ol – see beta sitosterol

A

A. byzantina – see avena sativa
A. diffusa – see avena sativa
Abobrinha do Mato – see cayaponia tayuya
Abromine – see betaine
Abufene – see beta alanine
Acidin-pepsin – see betaine
Adehl – see forskolin
Agarikusutake – see agaricus
Agathosma betulina – see buchu
Agathosma crenulata – see buchu
Agmathine – see agmatine
Agmatine sulfate – see agmatine
Agnus castus – see chasteberry
Almond Mushroom – see agaricus

Alpha Glycerol Phosphoryl Choline – see alpha glycerylphosphorycholine
Alpha-aminovaleric acid – see norvaline
Alpha-GPC – see alpha glycerylphosphorycholine
Alpha-ketoglutarate – see alpha-ketoglutarate
Alpha-ketoglutaric acid – see alpha-ketoglutarate
alpha-Linolenate – see flaxseed oil
alpha-Linolenic acid – see flaxseed oil
alpha-Lnn – see flaxseed oil
Amachazuru – see gynostemma
Anapinta – see cayaponia tayuya
Andrestenol – see DHEA
Androstenolone – see DHEA
Angelicin – see beta sitosterol
Anhalin – see hordenine
Anhaline – see hordenine
Antagonil – see yohimbe
Aphrodine – see yohimbe
Arbutin – see uva ursi
Arctic root – see rhodiola rosea
Arctostaphylos uva ursi – see uva ursi
Argmatine – see agmatine
Aspartic acid D-form – see sodium d-aspartate
Aspartic acid, D- – see sodium d-aspartate
Asthisamhrta – see cissus quadrangularis
Aurantiin – see naringin
Avena Fructus – see avena sativa
Avenae herba – see avena sativa
Avenae stramentum – see avena sativa

B

Bacopa Monnieri – see bacopa monniera
Balsamodendrum mukul – see guggulsterones E & Z
Balsamodendrum wightii – see guggulsterones E & Z
Barosma betulina – see buchu

Barosma crenulata – see buchu
Barosma serratifolia – see buchu
Batavia Cassia – see cassia cinnamon
Bear's grape – see uva ursi
Bearberry – see uva ursi
Benphothiamine – see benfotiamine
Benzenecarbothioic acid S-[2-[[(4-amino-2-methyl-5-pyrimidinyl)methyl] formylamino]-1-[2-(phosphonooxy)ethyl]-1-propenyl] ester – see benfotiamine
Berberine sulfate – see berberine
Beta-Glycyrrhetic acid – see glycyrrhetinic acid
Beta-Glycyrrhetinic acid – see glycyrrhetinic acid
Beta-Glycyrrhetinic acid – see glycyrrhetinic acid
Betaine anhydrous – see betaine
Beta-phenyl-GABA – see phenibut
Beta-phenyl-gamma-aminobutyric acid – see phenibut
Betivina – see benfotiamine
Bilineurine – see choline
Biosone – see glycyrrhetinic acid
Biotamin – see benfotiamine
Boforsin – see forskolin
Bovinic acid – see conjugated linoleic acid
Brahmi – see bacopa monniera
Branched chain amino acids – see BCAAs
Brazil Mushroom – see agaricus
Brazilian cocoa – see guarana
Brindall berry – see HCA
Brindleberry – see HCA
Bryonia tayuya – see cayaponia tayuya
Bucco – see buchu
Bucku – see buchu
Bushman's hat – see hoodia

C

Cactine – see hordenine

Cafeina – see caffeine

Calcium β-Hydroxy β-Methylbutyrate Monohydrate – see HMB

Calcium Alpha-Ketoglutarate – see alpha-ketoglutarate

Calcium Glucarate – see calcium d-glucarate

Calcium-D Glucarate – see calcium d-glucarate

Calcium-D-Glucarate – see calcium d-glucarate

Caltrop – see tribulus terrestris

Camellia sinensis – see green tea

Cankerwort – see dandelion

Canton cassia – see cassia cinnamon

Capsicum – see capsaicin

Capsicutin – see capsaicin

Carpopogon pruriens – see mucuna pruriens

Cassia – see cassia cinnamon

Cassia aromaticum – see cassia cinnamon

Cassia bark – see cassia cinnamon

Cat's head – see tribulus terrestris

Cayaponia piauhiensis – see cayaponia tayuya

Cayenne pepper – see capsaicin

Chaste tree – see chasteberry

Chilli pepper – see capsaicin

Chinese cinnamon – see cassia cinnamon

Chinese Dodder – see dodder

Chinese sage – see danshen

Chirchita – see achyranthes

Choline Alfoscerate – see alpha glycerylphosphorycholine

Choline Bitartrate – see choline

Choline Chloride – see choline

Choline Citrate – see choline

Cholinum – see choline

Chromic Chloride – see chromium

Chromium Acetate – see chromium

Chromium Chloride – see chromium

Chromium III – see chromium

Chromium Nicotinate – see chromium

Chromium Picolinate – see chromium
Chromium Polynicotinate – see chromium
Chromium Trichloride – see chromium
Chromium Tripicolinate – see chromium
Cinchol – see beta sitosterol
Cinnamomum aromaticum – see cassia cinnamon
Cinnamomum cassia – see cassia cinnamon
Cis-9,trans-11 conjugated linoleic acid – see conjugated linoleic acid
Civamide – see capsaicin
CLA-Triacylglycerol – see conjugated linoleic acid
Coffeine – see caffeine
Cogumelo de Deus – see agaricus
Cogumelo do Sol – see agaricus
Coleonol – see forskolin
Coleus – see forskolin
Coleus barbatus – see forskolin
Coleus Forskohlii – see forskolin
Colforsin – see forskolin
Colforsina – see forskolin
Colforsine – see forskolin
Colforsinum – see forskolin
Commiphora Mukul – see guggulsterones E & Z
Commiphora wightii – see guggulsterones E & Z
Common bearberry – see uva ursi
Common hop – see humulus lupus
Corylopsin – see bergenin
Corynine – see yohimbe
Cowhage – see mucuna pruriens
Cow-Itch Plant – see mucuna pruriens
Creatin – see creatine monohydrate
Crepe Myrtle – see banaba
Cupreol – see beta sitosterol
Cuscuta – see dodder
Cuscuta chinensis – see dodder
Cuscuta epithymum – see dodder

Cuscutae – see dodder
Cuscutin – see bergenin

D

DADAVIT ® – see sodium d-aspartate
Damiana Aphrodisiaca – see damiana
Damiana de Guerrero – see damiana
Dan Shen – see danshen
D-Aspartate – see sodium d-aspartate
D-Aspartic acid – see sodium d-aspartate
Deer nut – see jojoba
Dehydroepiandrosterone – see DHEA
Dehydroisoandrosterone – see DHEA
Devil's horn – see tribulus terrestris
Devil's weed – see tribulus terrestris
Devil's guts – see dodder
Devil's hair – see dodder
D-glucaro-1,4-lactone (1,4 GL) – see calcium d-glucarate
D-glucofuranurono-6,3-lactone – see glucuronolactone
D-Glucuronic acid γ-lactone – see glucuronolactone
D-Glucuronolactone – see glucuronolactone
Diandron – see DHEA
Diandrone – see DHEA
Dicurone – see glucuronolactone
Diffusa aphrodisiaca – see damiana
Dimethylamylamine – see geranamine
Diosma betulina – see buchu
Divanillyltetrahydrofuran – see nettle
DMAA – see geranamine
Dodder seed – see dodder
Dolichos pruriens – see mucuna pruriens
Dungkulcha – see gynostemma

E

Ecdisten – see ecdysteroids
Ecdisteron – see ecdysteroids
Ecdysone – see ecdysteroids
Ecdysterone – see ecdysteroids
Ectysterone – see ecdysteroids
EGCG – see green tea
Eicosanetetraenoic acid – see arachidonic acid
Enoxolone – see glycyrrhetinic acid
Epigallocatechin gallate – see green tea
Epigallocatechin-3-gallate – see green tea
Eremursine – see hordenine
Evodia – see evodiamine
Evodia Lepta – see evodiamine
Evodia officinalis – see evodiamine
Evodia rutaecarpa – see evodiamine
Evodia rutaecarpa Bentham – see evodiamine
Evodiae – see evodiamine

F

Fairy herb – see gynostemma
Fenibut – see phenibut
Fenigam – see phenibut
Fenigama – see phenibut
Flax seed oil – see flaxseed oil
Forskholin – see forskolin
Forthane – see geranamine
Frambinone – see raspberry ketones
Fufang Danshen – see danshen

G

Garcinia acid – see HCA
Garcinia Cambogia – see HCA

Garcinia gummi-guta – see HCA
Garcinia Quaesita – see HCA
Geranium – see geranamine
Glucoxy – see glucuronolactone
Glucurolactona – see glucuronolactone
Glucurolactone – see glucuronolactone
Glucuron – see glucuronolactone
Glucurone – see glucuronolactone
Glucuronosan – see glucuronolactone
Gluronsan – see glucuronolactone
Glyccyrhetic acid – see glycyrrhetinic acid
Glycero-3-Phosphocholine – see alpha glycerylphosphorycholine
Glycerophosphocholine – see alpha glycerylphosphorycholine
Glycine betaine – see betaine
Glycocoll betaine – see betaine
Glycylbetaine – see betaine
Glycyrrhetic acid – see glycyrrhetinic acid
Glycyrrhetin – see glycyrrhetinic acid
Glycyrrhizic Acid – see glycyrrhetinic acid
Glycyrrhizinic acid – see glycyrrhetinic acid
Goat nut – see jojoba
Golden root – see rhodiola rosea
Goldthread – see dodder
Green tea catechins – see green tea
Guarana bread – see guarana
Guaranine – see caffeine
Guggul – see guggulsterones E & Z
Guggul Gum – see guggulsterones E & Z
Guggul Lipids – see guggulsterones E & Z
Guronsan – see glucuronolactone
Gynostemma pedatum – see gynostemma
Gynostemma pentaphyllum – see gynostemma

H

Hadjod – see cissus quadrangularis
Hadjora – see cissus quadrangularis
Hailweed – see dodder
Harbhanga – see cissus quadrangularis
Harzol – see beta sitosterol
Hasjora – see cissus quadrangularis
Herba Taraxaci – see dandelion
Herpestis monniera – see bacopa monniera
Himematsutake – see agaricus
HL-362 – see forskolin
Hoodia Gordonii – see hoodia
Hoodia Pilifera – see hoodia
Hops – see humulus lupus
Hordenin – see hordenine
Hydroxycitrate – see HCA
Hydroxycitric acid – see HCA
Hydroxymethylbutyrate – see HMB

I

Icosa-5,8,11,14-tetraenoic acid – see arachidonic acid
Indian Bdellium – see guggulsterones E & Z
Indian Pennywort – see bacopa monniera
Isodecanoic acid vanillylamide – see capsaicin
Isoinokosterone – see ecdysteroids

J

Jalanimba – see bacopa monniera
Jiao Chu Lan – see gynostemma
Jiao Gu Lan – see gynostemma
Jioagulan – see gynostemma
Johimbi – see yohimbe
Jojoba Meal – see jojoba

Jortaine – see betaine

K

Kawariharatake – see agaricus
Koffein – see caffeine
Kreatin – see creatine monohydrate
Krebiozon – see creatine monohydrate

L

L-75-1362B – see forskolin
Lagerstroemia speciosa – see banaba
L-alpha-Glycerophosphocholine – see alpha
glycerylphosphorycholine
L-alpha-Glycerophosphorylcholine – see alpha
glycerylphosphorycholine
L-Choline – see choline
Leontodon taraxacum – see dandelion
Linolenate – see flaxseed oil
Linolenic acid – see flaxseed oil
Linum crepitans – see flaxseed oil
Linum humile – see flaxseed oil
Linus usitatissimum – see flaxseed oil
Lion's tooth – see dandelion
L-norvaline – see norvaline
Longifolia jack – see eurycomia longifolia
Longjack – see eurycomia longifolia
L-ornithine alpha-ketoglutarate – see ornithine alpha-
ketoglutarate
L-Ornithine, N5-(aminocarbonyl)-, mono(+-)-
hydroxybutanedioate – see citrulline malate
Lupulin – see humulus lupus
Lupulinum – see humulus lupus
Lupulus – see humulus lupus
Lycine – see betaine

M

Malabar tamarind – see HCA
Malaysian Ginseng – see eurycomia longifolia
Mandelpilz – see agaricus
Mang Jing Zi – see chasteberry
Marian Thistle – see milk thistle
Mateina – see caffeine
Methoxyflavone – see methoxyisoflavone
methylaminomethyl 4-hydroxyphenyl carbinol – see synephrine
Methylated phosphatidylethanolamine – see choline
Methylglycocyamine – see creatine monohydrate
Methylhexaneamine – see geranamine
Methyltheobromine – see caffeine
Mexican damiana – see damiana
Mexican holly – see damiana
Milk soluble proteins – see whey protein
Miracle grass – see gynostemma
Moniera cuneifolia – see bacopa monniera
Monk's pepper – see chasteberry
Mucuna aterrima – see mucuna pruriens
Mucuna cochinchinensis – see mucuna pruriens
Mucuna prurita – see mucuna pruriens

N

N-(Aminoiminomethyl)-N-methylglycine – see creatine monohydrate
N,N-Dimethyltyramine – see hordenine
n-3 Fatty Acid – see flaxseed oil
N-4-aminobutylguanidine – see agmatine
N-amidinosarcosine – see creatine monohydrate
Naringenin-7-rhamnoglucoside – see naringin
Naringoside – see naringin
Nitanevril – see benfotiamine

Niu Xi – see achyranthes
N-methyl-N-guanylglycine – see creatine monohydrate
Norsympatol – see octopamine
Norsynephrine – see octopamine

O

Oat – see avena sativa
Octapamine – see octopamine
Octopaminum – see octopamine
Ocufors – see forskolin
OKG – see ornithine alpha-ketoglutarate
Oleoresin Capsicum – see capsaicin
Oleuroperin – see oleuropein
Oleurpein – see oleuropein
Omega-3 Fatty Acid – see flaxseed oil
Ornithine ketoglutarate – see ornithine alpha-ketoglutarate
Ornithine oxoglutarate – see ornithine alpha-ketoglutarate
Orpin rose – see rhodiola rosea
Oxedrine – see synephrine
Oxoglutaric acid – see alpha-ketoglutarate
Oxyneurine – see betaine
Oxyphenylon – see raspberry ketones

P

p-(2-Dimethylaminoethyl)phenol – see hordenine
Padang-Cassia – see cassia cinnamon
Paprika – see capsaicin
Parapetalifera betulina – see buchu
Parapetalifera crenulata – see buchu
Pasak bumi – see eurycomia longifolia
Paullinia cupana – see guarana
Pausinystalia yohimbe – see yohimbe
Payong ali – see eurycomia longifolia
Peltophorin – see bergenin

Penawar bias – see eurycomia longifolia
Penawar pahit – see eurycomia longifolia
Penta tea – see gynostemma
Pentylamine, 1,3-dimethyl- – see geranamine
Peyocactine – see hordenine
Phenigam – see phenibut
Phenigama – see phenibut
Phenigamma – see phenibut
Phenylgamma – see phenibut
Phosphocasein – see micellar casein
p-hydroxybutanone – see raspberry ketones
p-hydroxy-N,N-dimethylphenethylamine – see hordenine
p-hydroxyphenylethanolamine – see octopamine
p-hydroxy-α-[(methylamino)methyl]benzyl alcohol – see synephrine
Phytoecdysone – see ecdysteroids
Phytoecdysteroid – see ecdysteroids
Pig nut – see jojoba
Pirandai – see cissus quadrangularis
Plectranthus barbatus – see forskolin
p-methylaminoethanolphenol – see synephrine
p-Norsynephrin – see octopamine
Prasterone – see DHEA
Pregna-4,17(20)-diene-3,16-dione – see guggulsterones E & Z
Prestara – see DHEA
Pride of India – see banaba
Protodioscin – see tribulus terrestris
Protodioscine – see tribulus terrestris
Psicosterone – see DHEA
p-Synephrine – see synephrine
Pu Gong Ying – see dandelion
Puncturevine – see tribulus terrestris
Pyrolysate – see creatine monohydrate

Q

Quebrachine – see yohimbe
Quebrachol – see beta sitosterol
Queens Crape Myrtle – see banaba
Queen's Flower – see banaba

R

R = glucose : ramnose (2:1) - 26-o-beta-1-glucopiranosil, 22-hydroxifurost-5-en-3-beta, 26-diol, 3-o-beta-diglucoramnoside – see tribulus terrestris
Radix Salviae miltiorrhiza – see danshen
Rasketone – see raspberry ketones
Rauwolfia – see yohimbe
Red pepper – see capsaicin
Red sage root – see danshen
Rhamnol – see beta sitosterol
Rheosmin – see raspberry ketones
Rhodiole Rougeatre – see rhodiola rosea
Rosenroot – see rhodiola rosea
Roseroot – see rhodiola rosea
Rumenic acid – see conjugated linoleic acid

S

S-[(Z)-2-[(4-amino-2-methylpyrimidin-5-yl)methyl-formylamino]-5- phosphonooxypent-2-en-3-yl] benzenecarbothioate – see benfotiamine
Sage tree hemp – see chasteberry
Salvia Miltiorrhiza – see danshen
S-benzoylthiamine O-monophosphate – see benfotiamine
Scaldweed – see dodder
Sedum rhodiola – see rhodiola rosea
Sedum rosea – see rhodiola rosea
Semen Cuscutae – see dodder

Sesame lignan – see sesamin/episesamin
Sesame seed – see sesamin/episesamin
Sesamum indicum – see sesamin/episesamin
Silibinin – see milk thistle
Silybin – see milk thistle
Silybum – see milk thistle
Silybum marianum – see milk thistle
Silymarin – see milk thistle
Simmondsia chinensis – see jojoba
Sitosterin – see beta sitosterol
SN-glycero-3-phosphocholine – see alpha glycerylphosphorycholine
Southern ginseng – see gynostemma
St. Mary Thistle – see milk thistle
Stimol – see citrulline malate
Stinging nettle – see nettle
Stizolobium aterrimum – see mucuna pruriens
Stizolobium pruriens – see mucuna pruriens
Strangleweed – see dodder
Synephrin – see synephrine

T

Tanshen – see danshen
Tan-Shen – see danshen
Taraxacum dens-leonis – see dandelion
Taraxacum officinale – see dandelion
Taraxacum palustre – see dandelion
Taraxacum vulgare – see dandelion
Thein – see caffeine
Theine – see caffeine
Thiobenzoic acid S-ester with N-[(4-amino-2-methyl-5-pyrimidinyl)methyl]-N-(4-hydroxy-2-mercapto-1-methyl-1-butenyl)formamide O-phosphate – see benfotiamine
Thyme-Leave Gratiola – see bacopa monniera
Tongkat ali – see eurycomia longifolia

Tongkat baginda – see eurycomia longifolia
trans – resveratrol – see resveratrol
Trans-10,cis-12 conjugated linoleic acid – see conjugated linoleic acid
Trans-8-methyl-N-vanillyl-6-nonenamide, N-(4-Hydroxy-3-methoxyphenyl)-8-methyl-non-trans-6-enamide – see capsaicin
(E)-N-[(4-hydroxy-3-methoxyphenyl)methyl]-8-methylnon-6-enamide – see capsaicin
Trans-dehydroandrosterone – see DHEA
Trianosperma ficifolia – see cayaponia tayuya
Triastonal – see beta sitosterol
Trimethylethanolamine – see choline
Trimethylglycine – see betaine
Trimethylglycocoll – see betaine
Trivalent Chromium – see chromium
Turkesteron – see ecdysteroids
Turkesterone – see ecdysteroids
Turnera aphrodisiaca – see damiana
Turnera diffusa – see damiana
Turnera microphylla – see damiana
Turnerae diffusae folium – see damiana
Turnerae Diffusae Herba – see damiana

U

Umbellatine – see berberine
Uralenic acid – see glycyrrhetinic acid
Urtica dioica – see nettle
Urtica urens – see nettle

V

Veldt-grape – see cissus quadrangularis
Velvet Bean – see mucuna pruriens
Vitanevril – see benfotiamine

Vitex – see chasteberry
Vitex agnus-castus – see chasteberry
Vitis pentaphylla – see gynostemma
Vitis quadrangularis – see cissus quadrangularis

W

Waterhyssop – see bacopa monniera
Winged treebine – see cissus quadrangularis
Wu-chu-yu – see evodiamine

X

Xiancao – see gynostemma

Y

Yohimbine hydrochloride – see yohimbe

Z

Zoom – see guarana

www.doctorpg.org

www.doctorpg.org